Non-Invasive Ventilation Made Simple

WJM Kinnear

Non-Invasive Ventilation Made Simple

2nd edition

WJM Kinnear

Copyright © WJM Kinnear, 2007

Second Edition 2014

Published by 5m Publishing
Benchmark House
8 Smithy Wood Drive
Sheffield
S35 1QN
United Kingdom

www.5mpublishing.com
books@5mpublishing.com

ISBN: 978-1-9104550-0-5

A CIP catalogue record for this book is available from the British Library.

Printed and bound in the UK

For Sue, Anne and Katie

Contents

Abbreviations

ADRT	advance decision to refuse treatment
AMU	acute medicine unit
ARDS	adult respiratory distress syndrome
ASB	assisted spontaneous breathing
AVAPS	average volume-assured pressure-support
BIPAP	bi-level positive airway pressure
BP	blood pressure
CF	cystic fibrosis
cmH_2O	centimetres of water
CO_2	carbon dioxide
COPD	chronic obstructive pulmonary disease
CPAP	continuous positive airway pressure
CSF	cerebrospinal fluid
CXR	chest X-ray
ED	emergency department
ENAP	expiratory negative airway pressure
EPAP	expiratory positive airway pressure
ET	endotracheal
FEV1	forced expired volume in one second
FRC	functional residual capacity
GCS	Glasgow Coma Scale
HDU	high dependency unit
HME	heat and moisture exchanger
ICU	intensive care unit
I:E	inspiratory:expiratory
IPAP	inspiratory positive airway pressure
IPPV	intermittent positive pressure ventilation
kPa	kilopascal

l	litre
LTOT	long-term oxygen therapy
LVF	left ventricular failure
MEP	maximum expiratory mouth pressure
MIP	maximum inspiratory mouth pressure
ml	millilitre
mmHg	millimetres of mercury
MND	motor neurone disease
NIV	non-invasive ventilation
O_2	oxygen
OHS	obesity-hypoventilation syndrome
OSA	obstructive sleep apnoea
$PaCO_2$	arterial partial pressure of carbon dioxide
PaO_2	arterial partial pressure of oxygen
PAO_2	alveolar partial pressure of oxygen
PCF	peak cough flow
PEEPi	intrinsic positive end-expiratory pressure
PEFR	peak expiratory flow rate
RCT	randomised controlled trial
RR	respiratory rate
SNIP	sniff nasal inspiratory pressure
SaO_2	arterial oxygen saturation
SARS	severe acute respiratory syndrome
SpO_2	peripheral oxygen saturation
TB	tuberculosis
VC	vital capacity
Vt	tidal volume

Key Terms

Alveolar hypoventilation: Reduced ventilation of the gas-exchanging part of the lungs, with inadequate elimination of CO_2.

Aspiration: Inhalation of gastric contents into the lungs.

Assist: When the ventilator helps the patient's spontaneous breathing pattern.

Autotriggering: Self-triggering of the ventilator to initiate a breath, usually caused by high flow of air down the circuit.

Bi-level positive airway pressure: The commonest mode of non-invasive ventilation, combining inspiratory and expiratory positive airway pressure.

Central hypoventilation: Type 2 respiratory failure caused by poor respiratory drive.

Control: When the ventilator delivers breaths to the patient independently of their breathing pattern.

Expiratory positive airway pressure: Positive pressure applied to the airway during expiration.

Fractional inspired oxygen: The concentration of oxygen a patient breathes in.

Hypercapnia: Elevated arterial carbon dioxide level.

Hypoxaemia: Low arterial oxygen level.

Inspiratory positive airway pressure: Positive pressure applied to the airway during inspiration.

Inspiratory:expiratory ratio: The ratio of the time spent in inspiration to that in expiration.

Interface: The device used to connect the ventilator to the patient.

Intrinsic positive end-expiratory pressure: Pressure inside the thorax when the lungs are unable to empty completely.

Intubation: Insertion of an endotracheal tube to provide "invasive" ventilation.

Non-invasive intermittent positive pressure ventilation: The commonest pressure-control mode of non-invasive ventilation.

Non-invasive ventilation: Artificial ventilation that doesn't use an endotracheal tube or tracheostomy.

Pressure-control ventilation: NIV where both the pressure and timing of breaths are set.

Pressure-support ventilation: NIV where only the pressure is set, the timing being determined by the patient's own breathing pattern.

Pressure-targeted ventilation: NIV where the target pressure for each breath is set.

Obesity-hypoventilation syndrome: Chronic type 2 respiratory failure in very obese patients.

Re-breathing: The patient inhales the air they have just breathed out.

Respiratory acidosis: Elevation of the $PaCO_2$ with a low pH level.

Rise time: The time taken at the start of inspiration to reach the target pressure.

Scoliosis: Curvature of the spine.

Span: The difference between IPAP and EPAP.

Tidal volume: The volume of air entering the lungs with each breath.

Type 1 respiratory failure: Failure of oxygenation, with a normal or low $PaCO_2$.

Type 2 respiratory failure: Failure of ventilation, with an elevated $PaCO_2$.

Vital capacity: The maximum amount of air a patient can take — or blow out — with a single breath.

Volume-targeted ventilation: NIV where the target tidal volume for each breath is set, rather than the pressure.

Weaning: The gradual reduction of ventilatory support until either the patient is breathing independently or further reduction cannot be achieved.

Work of breathing: The amount of energy used in moving air in and out of the lungs.

1
Background

Learning points

By the end of this chapter you should be able to:

- Describe the difference between non-invasive ventilation (NIV) and invasive ventilation
- List a few different places where NIV might be used
- Explain why you think you need to know about NIV
- Give a few examples of patients who might need NIV acutely in hospital, or long-term at home

What is ventilation?

When we talk about a patient being ventilated, we usually mean artificial ventilation provided by a life-support machine or ventilator. (Sometimes this is called "mechanical ventilation".) The main aim of ventilation is to get air in and out of the lungs.

When you blow up a balloon, you apply a positive pressure to the opening to inflate it (Figure 1.1). The positive pressure might come from your breathing muscles, a cylinder of pressurised gas, a blower or a piston-style pump like a bicycle pump. Mechanical ventilators are also basically sources of positive pressure — apply a positive pressure to the airway and the lungs will inflate; take the pressure away and they will deflate. We'll spend quite a lot of time talking about different ways of using this "positive airway pressure".

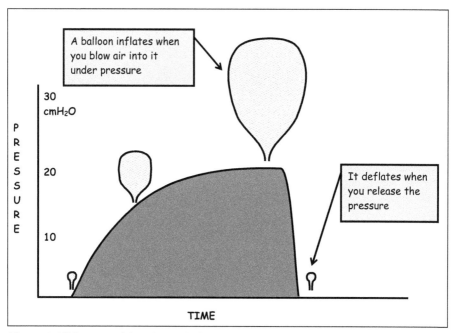

Figure 1.1 When you blow into a balloon, the positive pressure you generate causes the balloon to inflate. When you take your mouth away, the pressure falls back to zero and the balloon deflates. This is the same principle as a non-invasive ventilator inflating the lungs.

What is non-invasive ventilation?

"Invasive" ventilation means the ventilator is connected to an endotracheal tube or tracheostomy tube, by-passing the upper airway and larynx.

"Non-invasive" ventilation means that the ventilator is attached to a mask which is placed on the face. There are a few other ways of providing artificial ventilation which are non-invasive — iron lungs, cuirasses, pneumobelts, rocking beds etc. Their use is now largely confined to specialist centres and we won't be discussing them further.

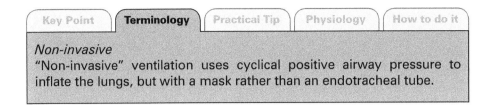

Non-invasive
"Non-invasive" ventilation uses cyclical positive airway pressure to inflate the lungs, but with a mask rather than an endotracheal tube.

Continuous positive airway pressure (CPAP) can be used to improve oxygenation, or to keep the upper airway patent. Although the same sort of mask is used, it is not really a form of ventilation.

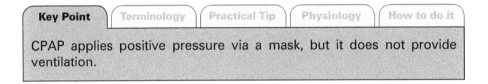

CPAP applies positive pressure via a mask, but it does not provide ventilation.

Why do I need to know about NIV?

- NIV has become the standard treatment for most patients with hypercapnic respiratory failure who need ventilatory support
- NIV is used on high dependency units (HDU), respiratory wards, acute medicine units (AMU) and in emergency departments (ED). If you work in any of these areas, you need to know about it
- On the intensive care unit (ICU), NIV is used as a primary treatment for respiratory failure and also to help wean from invasive ventilation. Even if you are fully conversant with the sorts of ventilators used for invasive ventilation, there are some important aspects of NIV which you need to understand
- For every 100,000 people in the population, there will be between 5 and 10 patients who use NIV at home, often just at night. They may develop acute respiratory failure for example when they get a chest infection — and need admission to hospital. You may also want to know more if you are likely to come across these patients in clinics or in the community

What do I need to know about NIV?

In terms of equipment, a ventilator is usually thought of as a piece of apparatus used in the operating theatre or on an ICU. It will have lots of control knobs and dials. The operation of these is best left to an anaesthetist or intensivist. Non-invasive ventilators are much simpler and easier to use than invasive ventilators. We'll work through how to set them up for different types of patient. The circuits and masks are also pretty straightforward.

Standard ICU ventilators tend not to be very good at NIV, because they were designed for use with an endotracheal tube and can't cope with the leaks that are inevitable with a mask. They are also much more complicated.

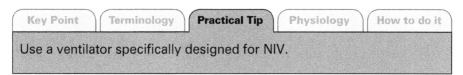

Key Point	Terminology	**Practical Tip**	Physiology	How to do it

Use a ventilator specifically designed for NIV.

As the years go by we are getting a clearer picture of which groups of patients get the most benefit from NIV. We'll look at each of these in turn.

We're also getting better at predicting the problems that occur during NIV. You'll learn how to prevent them or sort them out.

These basic topics form several themes that run through this book: the equipment you need for NIV, the patients you will be treating, "how to do it" and the underlying physiological principles.

How should I use this book?

Everything you need to know should be included at some point. At the start of each chapter there is an indication in **Learning points** of what is covered.

I have worked on the assumption that you are likely to read through this book once, then come back to it for reference. The technical, clinical and theoretical topics are mixed together, in the hope of an easier and more enjoyable read. It should still be simple to refer back to a particular topic.

In this chapter you have already come across index cards with *Key points, Practical tips* and *Terminology*. The other highlighted sections are *How to do it* and *Physiology*.

Key Point | Terminology | Practical Tip | **Physiology** | How to do it

Pressure and volume

When you blow up a balloon, if you blow harder (i.e. use a higher pressure) then the balloon will inflate more (i.e. increase in volume). The same principle applies to the lungs: using a higher positive airway pressure will increase lung volume (Figure 1.2).

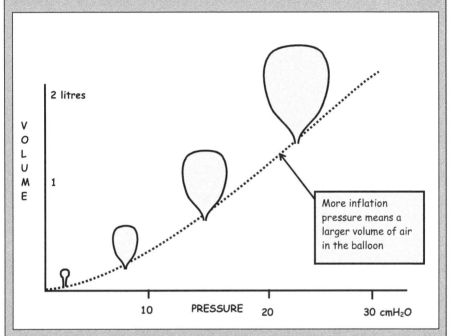

Figure 1.2 When you blow up a balloon, the more pressure you use, the bigger the balloon gets. The same principle applies to the lungs with non-invasive ventilation: more pressure means more volume.

Even at the end of expiration the lungs are still partially inflated, so we don't encounter the difficult bit that occurs right at the start of blowing up a balloon. With our lungs, however, it does become harder and harder to get more air in as the volume increases. The pressure-volume curve of the lungs is just that: a curve not a straight line. For any given increase in positive airway pressure during NIV, the change in volume is less at higher lung volumes (Figure 1.3).

cont ...

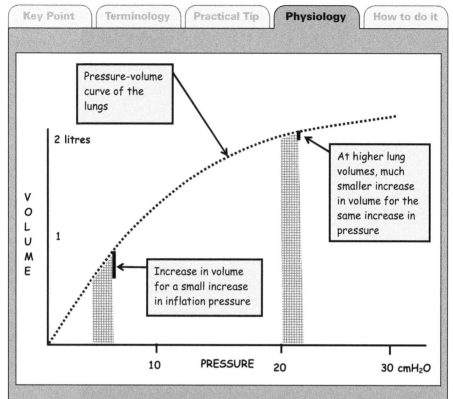

Figure 1.3 Pressure-volume curve of the lungs. At higher lung volumes, for a given change in positive airway pressure the change in volume of the lungs is less.

Summary

- NIV is artificial ventilation using a mask rather than an endotracheal tube
- NIV is used widely in many different acute situations — you need to know something about it if you work in an acute hospital
- NIV is much simpler to manage than invasive ventilation on ICU
- Quite a few patients use NIV at home, often just at night

2
Building Blocks

Learning points

By the end of this chapter you should be able to:

- Draw a block diagram showing the three main components of NIV
- Explain why mask leaks are such a problem

A patient with an exacerbation of their chronic obstructive pulmonary disease (COPD) comes into hospital with acute hypercapnic respiratory failure. They aren't improving despite optimal drug therapy and controlled oxygen. You decide they need NIV: you will need a pump (the ventilator), an interface (the mask) and tubing to connect the two together (the circuit), as shown in Figure 2.1.

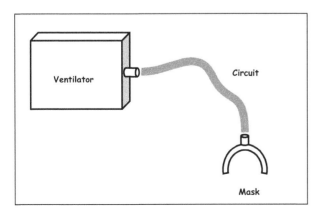

Figure 2.1 The three components of NIV: a ventilator, connected by circuit tubing to a mask.

This sort of set-up may look familiar to you if you see patients with obstructive sleep apnoea (OSA) on CPAP: they have a blower, tube and mask. The pressure is continuous so a graph of pressure versus time will be a straight line (Figure 2.2).

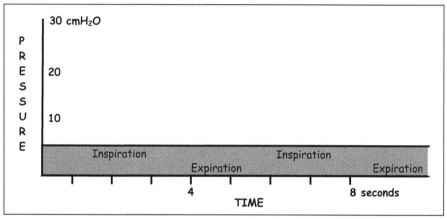

Figure 2.2 Pressure-time trace of CPAP. Positive airway pressure is applied continuously, with no variation between inspiration and expiration.

CPAP is used just to keep the upper airway open. For NIV, we want to get air in and out of the lungs as well, so we'll need to vary the pressure up and down (Figure 2.3).

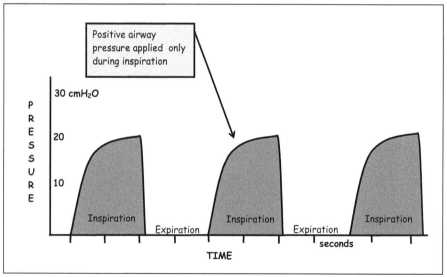

Figure 2.3 Pressure-time trace of NIV. Positive airway pressure is applied during inspiration only. (This is intermittent positive pressure ventilation, or IPPV – we'll often add a bit of pressure in expiration as well, but more of this later.)

The pump

The pump is a simple piece of equipment which contains a fan (or sometimes bellows) to deliver air to the patient. There are different ways of setting up the pump – we will discuss these in detail later on. All we need for the moment is something that will deliver air under positive pressure. We won't spend time looking at individual makes of ventilator, as new designs come along every year.

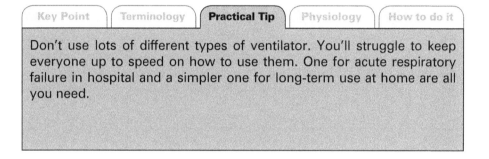

Key Point | Terminology | **Practical Tip** | Physiology | How to do it

Don't use lots of different types of ventilator. You'll struggle to keep everyone up to speed on how to use them. One for acute respiratory failure in hospital and a simpler one for long-term use at home are all you need.

The circuit

The circuit is also simple — a length of tubing usually about a metre or so long. It needs to be long enough to allow the patient to move around in bed; if it is too long then the ventilator may struggle with the resistance to flow. The tube should be wide bore to allow the air to flow freely into the patient — about 22 mm in diameter, similar to the "elephant" tubing you may have used to deliver high-flow oxygen on the wards. Tubing with a smooth internal surface offers the least resistance to flow, but corrugated tubing is fine for most NIV purposes. (It needs to be strong enough not to collapse when something is put on top of it.)

You will also probably know from setting up CPAP that you need a hole somewhere in the circuit, to allow the exhaled air to escape. If we didn't have an expiratory port, our patient would end up re-breathing "stale" air containing carbon dioxide and not much oxygen (Figure 2.4).

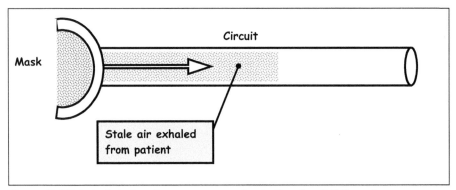

Figure 2.4 Exhaled air, low in oxygen, remains in the circuit if there is no exhalation port or valve.

Without an exhalation valve or port, NIV would just push the exhaled air (which doesn't have much oxygen left in it) back into the patient (Figure 2.5).

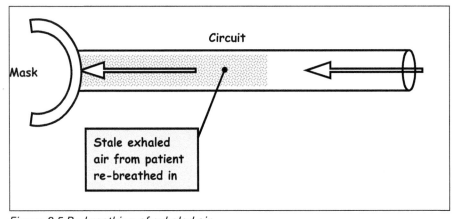

Figure 2.5 Re-breathing of exhaled air.

How we decide on expiratory holes and valves will depend upon the way we use NIV, but we'll discuss these later. In essence, the circuit is a wide bore tube which takes the air from the ventilator to the patient.

The mask

The mask is the crucial thing about NIV. Getting a mask to fit well is the most skilful bit. It needs to be comfortable for the patient. There must be a good enough seal so that most of the air from the ventilator goes into the patient rather than leaking around the edges of the mask.

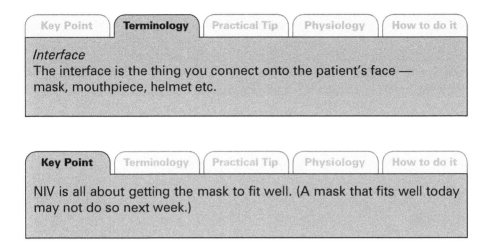

Terminology

Interface
The interface is the thing you connect onto the patient's face — mask, mouthpiece, helmet etc.

Key Point

NIV is all about getting the mask to fit well. (A mask that fits well today may not do so next week.)

Leaks

The main problem with NIV is managing leaks. You will spend a lot of time adjusting masks to try and minimise leaks. Leaks mean that ventilators have to work harder to get the mask up to the required pressure, they don't know how much of the air they delivered in a breath has gone into the patient and how much has leaked into the room (which is why we tend not to use ventilators on which we only set the volume of each breath, or tidal volume) and it is more difficult for them to work out when the patient wants to breathe.

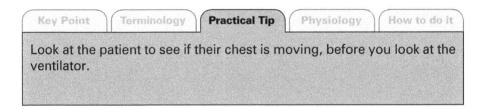

Practical Tip

Look at the patient to see if their chest is moving, before you look at the ventilator.

During sleep, leaks around the mask and through the mouth are the main reason that nocturnal hypoventilation persists despite NIV. Air leaking around the mask blows into the patient's eyes, makes a noise and is generally uncomfortable.

Key Point | **Terminology** | Practical Tip | Physiology | How to do it

PaO_2 and $PaCO_2$

NIV is used to treat respiratory failure. To decide whether or not a patient is in respiratory failure, we need to know about their oxygen and carbon dioxide levels. This usually requires an arterial blood gas sample, on which we measure the amount of oxygen (PO_2) and carbon dioxide (PCO_2). The "P" stands for partial pressure and for blood gases we put in "a" to indicate "arterial", hence PaO_2 and $PaCO_2$. (A capital "A" is used for alveolar, as we'll see later on.)

Key Point | Terminology | Practical Tip | **Physiology** | How to do it

Oxygen cascade

Atmospheric pressure is around 100 kPa, and air contains 21% oxygen. The part of atmospheric pressure which is attributed to oxygen (partial pressure) is therefore 21 kPa.

When we inspire, our upper airways humidify the dry air. The water vapour takes up about 6 kPa of pressure, so in the lungs PO_2 is 21% of 94 rather than 21% of 100 kPa. This is 20 kPa, or near enough.

If the air we breathe in has a PO_2 of 20 kPa, why isn't our PaO_2 that high? (The normal range for PaO_2 is 10-13 kPa). There are two reasons for this discrepancy. Firstly, some of the available space for gas is taken up by CO_2 — let's say about another 6 kPa (i.e. roughly the same as $PaCO_2$). That takes us down from 20 to 14 kPa.

If alveolar PO_2 (called PAO_2) is 14 kPa, there is then a slight fall across the alveolar-capillary membrane, perhaps 1 kPa in a normal subject breathing air. (This is called the A-a gradient.) One less than 14 is 13, the top end of our normal range for PaO_2 (Figure 2.6).

(Loss of lung surface area for gas exchange makes the A-a gradient a bit larger, which is why the "normal" value for an elderly patient may be as low as 10 kPa.)

cont ...

Key Point | Terminology | Practical Tip | **Physiology** | How to do it

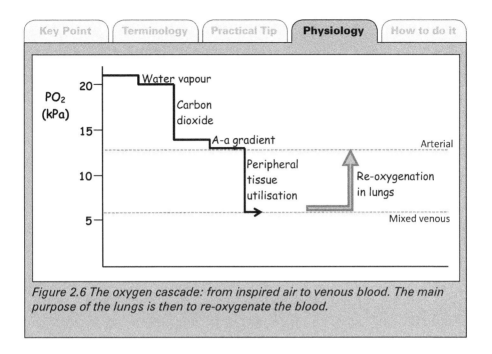

Figure 2.6 The oxygen cascade: from inspired air to venous blood. The main purpose of the lungs is then to re-oxygenate the blood.

Summary

- NIV uses an air pump (ventilator), connected by a tube (circuit) to a mask (interface)
- Fitting the mask is the skilful bit

3
Basic Principles

Learning points

By the end of this chapter you should be able to:

- Draw a graph showing how airway pressure increases and decreases during NIV
- Explain how this produces tidal volume
- Compute minute ventilation from tidal volume and breathing frequency

Thinking again of the lung as a balloon, to expand it in the way that NIV expands the chest, we need to blow air in. Imagine blowing into the balloon, and then taking your mouth away to let the air flow out again as the balloon collapses — for the sake of simplicity, this is a very small balloon that you can blow up in one breath. If we measured the pressure in the balloon as you blew into it, there would be a positive pressure, say 15 cmH$_2$O. When you took your mouth away, the balloon would deflate and the pressure would return to zero (atmospheric). This is the principle of NIV, except that instead of you blowing up a balloon there is a ventilator blowing air into a patient.

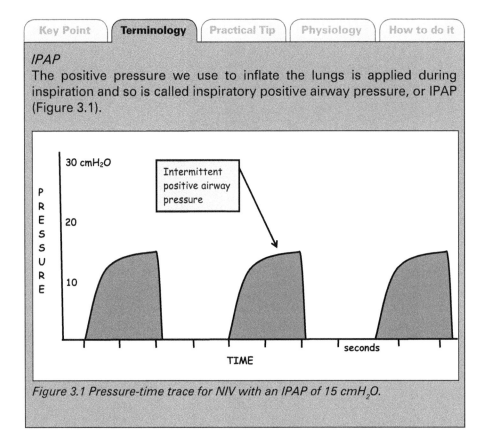

| Key Point | **Terminology** | Practical Tip | Physiology | How to do it |

IPAP

The positive pressure we use to inflate the lungs is applied during inspiration and so is called inspiratory positive airway pressure, or IPAP (Figure 3.1).

Figure 3.1 Pressure-time trace for NIV with an IPAP of 15 cmH$_2$O.

Ventilation

The volume of air entering the lungs with each breath is called the tidal volume (Vt). If we look again at the pressure-volume curve of the lungs (Figure 3.2), IPAP inflates the lungs by moving them further up the curve. Releasing the pressure allows them to return to their resting volume. The higher the IPAP you use, the greater the Vt you will get.

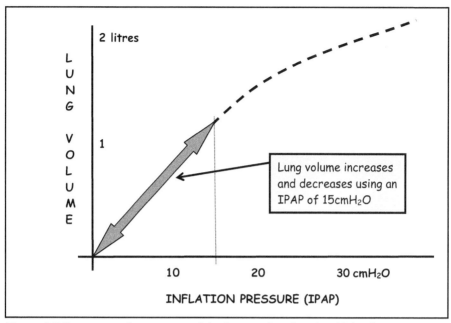

Figure 3.2 Pressure-volume curve of the lungs, showing the tidal volume obtained with an IPAP of 15 cmH$_2$O.

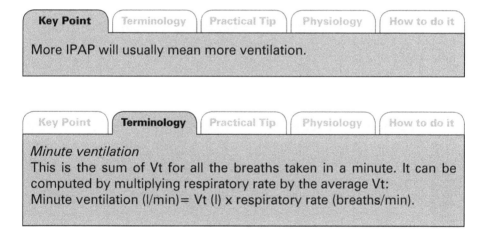

Key Point	Terminology	Practical Tip	Physiology	How to do it

More IPAP will usually mean more ventilation.

Key Point	**Terminology**	Practical Tip	Physiology	How to do it

Minute ventilation
This is the sum of Vt for all the breaths taken in a minute. It can be computed by multiplying respiratory rate by the average Vt:
Minute ventilation (l/min)= Vt (l) x respiratory rate (breaths/min).

Leak compensation

NIV ventilators are built to cope with leaks. They just blow harder to keep the IPAP to where we want it to be. We have set a target for IPAP, and the ventilator's job is to maintain that pressure target.

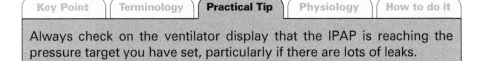

| Key Point | Terminology | Practical Tip | Physiology | How to do it |

Pressure-targeted ventilation
In the example we used earlier in this chapter, we aimed for a pressure of 15 cmH$_2$O. This is the target pressure which we set on the ventilator. Most NIV involves pressure-targeted modes.

Obviously at some stage the leak will be too much for the ventilator to cope with: if you take the mask off the patient, there will be a massive "leak" and the IPAP will fall way below where we want it to be. Modern NIV machines cope with pretty much anything short of taking the mask off.

| Key Point | Terminology | Practical Tip | Physiology | How to do it |

Always check on the ventilator display that the IPAP is reaching the pressure target you have set, particularly if there are lots of leaks.

Summary

- **NIV uses positive pressure to push air into the chest**
- **This is like blowing up a balloon**
- **Higher pressures generate larger volumes**

4
Scoliosis

Learning points

By the end of this chapter you should be able to:

*   Describe how scoliosis affects breathing
*   Identify which patients with scoliosis need NIV

Let's take a short break from the nuts and bolts of ventilation and look at a clinical condition. Patients with scoliosis account for only a small proportion of those using NIV, but the principles of how to set them up on a ventilator are fairly straightforward and will serve well to illustrate some important concepts.

Spinal curvature

There are two types of spinal curvature — kyphosis and scoliosis. In kyphosis the spine is curved in only one plane, front to back. If you look from the side (or on a lateral chest X-ray) the spine is curved forward, but if you look from the front or back the spine doesn't curve to one side or the other. Kyphosis has to be very severe to result in ventilatory failure, because the orientation of the ribs and the diaphragm remain fairly normal.

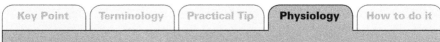

Key Point	Terminology	Practical Tip	Physiology	How to do it

Kyphosis (antero-posterior curvature of the spine) is only rarely the explanation for why a patient has slipped into respiratory failure.

Scoliosis involves rotation of the spine, which looks curved if you view from either the side or the back. When the thoracic spine is scoliotic, the ribs are very distorted. The mechanics of breathing are affected much more severely than in kyphosis.

Key Point	Terminology	Practical Tip	**Physiology**	How to do it

Load and capacity
The job of the inspiratory muscles is to pump air into the lungs, in other words to provide ventilation.

Inadequate ventilation may occur if the inspiratory muscles are weak, as we'll see when we look at muscular dystrophies, or if the work they have to do to expand the lungs is just too much for them. This balance, between the work required to be done and the strength available to do it, is often referred to as load and capacity. You can think of it as a set of scales (Figure 4.1).

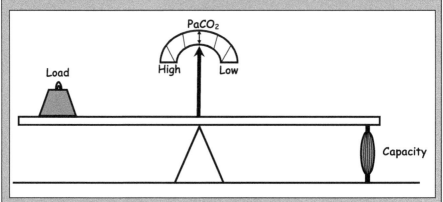

Figure 4.1 If load and capacity are evenly matched, the scales remain more or less level, with the pointer in the normal range.

cont ...

Key Point   Terminology   Practical Tip   **Physiology**   How to do it

In scoliosis the inspiratory muscles are fine, the main problem is that the weight is too great, so the scales tip over and the dial shows a higher $PaCO_2$. The load on the inspiratory muscles is too much for them to maintain adequate ventilation (Figure 4.2).

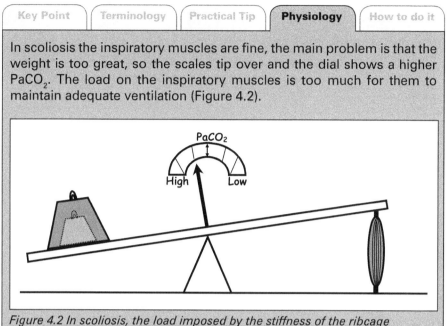

Figure 4.2 In scoliosis, the load imposed by the stiffness of the ribcage exceeds the capacity of the inspiratory muscles. The scales tip over and the result is a high $PaCO_2$ (hypercapnia).

Ventilatory failure in scoliosis

If the spinal curvature is more than a right angle, then there is a significant risk that the patient will develop respiratory problems at some stage. The vital capacity (VC) of these patients is almost always less than 50% predicted. (Remember to use arm span to estimate height: real height will be lower because of the spinal curvature, so you would come up with smaller predicted lung volumes.)

Key Point   Terminology   **Practical Tip**   Physiology   How to do it

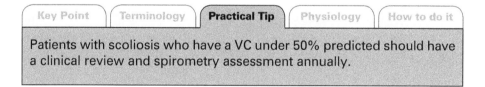

Patients with scoliosis who have a VC under 50% predicted should have a clinical review and spirometry assessment annually.

There are a few other risk factors for respiratory failure:

- **If the patient has ever had spinal surgery then they are less likely to slip into respiratory failure, possibly because the spine is more stable**
- **If the scoliosis was present before the patient was five years old, then they will not have developed the normal complement of alveoli and are more likely to develop respiratory failure. (Patients with congenital scoliosis should have an echocardiogram to check for associated cardiac defects)**
- **If the scoliosis is the result of weakness of the paraspinal muscles — from polio or muscular dystrophy — there will usually be associated respiratory muscle weakness and respiratory failure is much more common**

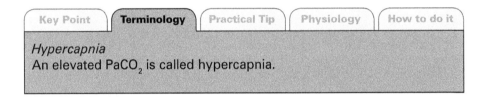

| Key Point | **Terminology** | Practical Tip | Physiology | How to do it |

Hypercapnia
An elevated $PaCO_2$ is called hypercapnia.

Once the daytime $PaCO_2$ is elevated, a crisis is just around the corner and the patient needs to be started on NIV; they may only need to have this at night, but they will need it for the rest of their lives. It doesn't matter what the pH is — the $PaCO_2$ will have been up for a while, and the kidneys will have retained bicarbonate to keep the amounts of acid and alkali ("base") in balance. The bottom line is that if the $PaCO_2$ is up, the load is too much for the respiratory muscles — they need help.

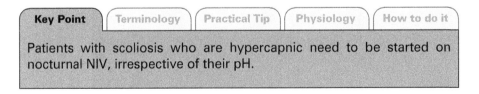

| **Key Point** | Terminology | Practical Tip | Physiology | How to do it |

Patients with scoliosis who are hypercapnic need to be started on nocturnal NIV, irrespective of their pH.

Resting the respiratory muscles at night leaves them with enough capacity to maintain adequate spontaneous ventilation during the day. The prognosis for patients with scoliosis on NIV is excellent, with five-year survival rates around 80%.

| Key Point | Terminology | **Practical Tip** | Physiology | How to do it |

Many patients with severe scoliosis will underventilate for short periods during rapid eye movement (REM) sleep. You don't need to start NIV if the patient has no symptoms of sleep disturbance, but review the patient every 6 or 12 months and undertake a sleep study annually.

Non-invasive ventilation

So, our patient with scoliosis has slipped into hypercapnic respiratory failure, because their respiratory muscles are tired from having had to work so hard to expand the distorted ribcage. The aim of NIV is to take over the work of breathing from the respiratory muscles, to give them a rest. Since the distorted ribcage is going to be pretty hard to inflate, we will need to use an IPAP of at least 20 cmH$_2$O to achieve adequate ventilation.

Let's choose a nasal mask — we'll be looking at the different options in the next chapter. To overcome the problem of re-breathing into the circuit, we'll put an expiratory valve next to the mask (Figure 4.3).

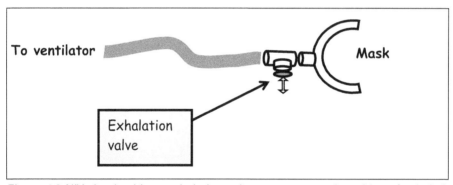

Figure 4.3 NIV circuit with an exhalation valve, to prevent re-breathing of exhaled air.

In this situation, we want to rest the respiratory muscles as much as we can. We don't want them to waste any energy triggering the ventilator. If we use enough IPAP to provide a reasonable Vt and set the respiratory rate so that the patient feels comfortable, they will hopefully relax and let the ventilator do all the work. To start with, the rate should be about the same as the patient's spontaneous respiratory rate. This is likely to be quite fast.

Key Point | Terminology | Practical Tip | Physiology | How to do it

When you start a patient with scoliosis or neuromuscular disease on NIV, set the ventilator rate to the patient's spontaneous breathing rate.

Key Point | Terminology | **Practical Tip** | Physiology | How to do it

On many ventilators the respiratory rate is always referred to as the back-up rate. In pressure-control modes, this is the actual rate of ventilation, not just the back-up.

In order to make the patient as comfortable as possible, set the length of inspiration to the same as their usual breathing pattern. Remember, we want them to relax and not to do any triggering. This mode of ventilation is called pressure-control: the ventilator determines the respiratory rate and the duration of inspiration. It works well for long-term ventilation, when we want to rest the respiratory muscles at night. It is also useful when the patient's own respiratory drive is too poor to rely on, for example in obesity-hypoventilation. We'll come back to all this later.

Key Point | **Terminology** | Practical Tip | Physiology | How to do it

Pressure-control
In pressure-control modes, the timing of breathing is controlled by the ventilator rather than the patient.

Key Point | Terminology | Practical Tip | Physiology | How to do it

Pressure-control mode is the best mode of ventilation for most patients using NIV at home.

Key Point | Terminology | Practical Tip | Physiology | **How to do it**

Start a patient with scoliosis on NIV
- Choose a mask
- Set up the circuit with an expiratory valve
- Count the patient's breathing rate
- Turn the ventilator on
- Set the ventilator rate to the patient's breathing rate
- Adjust the timing of the ventilator so that the inspiration and expiration are approximately the same as the patient's own spontaneous breaths
- Set the IPAP to 20 cmH$_2$O
- Hold the mask on the patient, and ask them to breathe in and out of the mask so they get used to the sensation of the pressure from the ventilator
- When they have grown accustomed to NIV, strap the mask in place
- Watch for a few minutes
- Adjust the mask to minimise leaks
- Adjust the pressure up or down, within the range 15-30 cmH$_2$O, to the lowest level that gives good chest expansion
- See if the patient feels comfortable with a slightly slower respiratory rate
- Write down the ventilator settings

Key Point | Terminology | Practical Tip | **Physiology** | How to do it

Compliance
We have already looked at the pressure-volume curve of the lungs. The slope of this curve gives us an idea of how difficult it is to get air into the lungs — a flatter slope means less volume for the same pressure change. The term for this is compliance. Strictly speaking this is the compliance of the whole respiratory system, both the lungs and the ribcage. Stiffness of either the lungs or the ribcage will reduce the total compliance (Figure 4.4). Although this is clearly a curve, traditionally compliance is taken as the slope of the line immediately above the resting end-expiratory position (a point known as functional residual capacity, or FRC).

cont ...

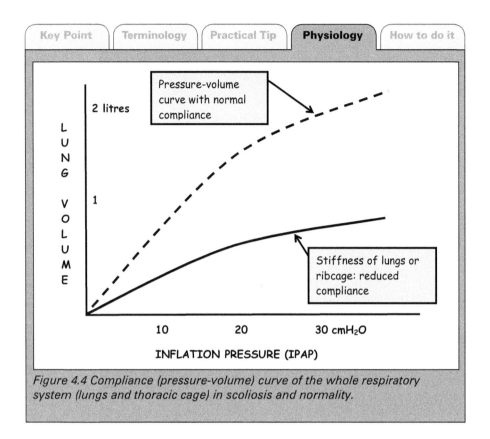

Figure 4.4 Compliance (pressure-volume) curve of the whole respiratory system (lungs and thoracic cage) in scoliosis and normality.

Summary

- Patients with scoliosis of sufficient severity to reduce VC below 50% predicted are at risk of hypercapnic respiratory failure
- If the daytime $PaCO_2$ is elevated, start long-term nocturnal NIV
- Use pressure-control NIV

5
Masks

Learning points

By the end of this chapter you should be able to:

- Decide whether to use a nasal or full-face mask for NIV
- Choose a mask of an appropriate size
- Demonstrate how you would fit the mask to the patient
- Explain when you would use other interfaces such as mouthpieces and helmets

The most crucial aspect of NIV is the "interface" between the ventilator and the patient. This is usually a mask, but there are a few other options to consider such as nasal pillows, mouthpieces and helmets.

Oro-nasal masks

If you get breathless, you tend to breathe through your mouth. For this reason, in most acute situations a mask which covers the nose and mouth is the best option to try first. The mask has a cushioned edge to form a seal with the face. You may need to try several sizes on the patient before you get the best fit. When you strap the mask in place, tighten the straps as tight as is necessary to prevent leaks — if this is intolerably tight for the patient, try a different size of mask. If this doesn't work, try a nasal mask.

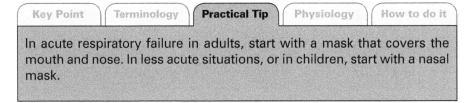

| Key Point | Terminology | Practical Tip | Physiology | How to do it |

NIV masks are very different from oxygen masks — they fit much more tightly to the face in order to achieve a seal.

Nasal masks

Face masks tend to move around a bit. This isn't surprising considering how mobile our jaws are. A nasal mask is much more stable on the bones of the face. For patients starting NIV in a non-acute setting, a nasal mask is often the best choice to try first. Smaller masks tend to work better than larger ones. Keep the patient's dentures in (unless their consciousness is impaired): the mask will tend to stay in place better.

| Key Point | Terminology | Practical Tip | Physiology | How to do it |

In acute respiratory failure in adults, start with a mask that covers the mouth and nose. In less acute situations, or in children, start with a nasal mask.

You might think that when a ventilator is attached to a mask over the nose, the air would come straight out of the mouth. In practice, patients quickly learn to use their soft palate to block off the connection between their nose and mouth, and the ventilator works fine. Some patients get the hang of this quite quickly, a few never manage it. Managing it all night is another matter.

Key Point | Terminology | Practical Tip | Physiology | **How to do it**

Reduce mask leaks
- Adjust the patient's head and neck to a "neutral" position, where they are well-centred in the bed with their head relaxed on their pillow
- Pull the mask slightly away from the face, centre it and "re-bed" it on the patient
- Press gently on the mask and see if this reduces the leak; if so, unclip the straps (lower ones first) and tighten them slightly; (over-tightening the straps makes the mask uncomfortable without reducing leakage much)
- Change to a smaller mask
- Try a different style of mask
- Try an individually moulded mask, if this is available
- Reduce the IPAP. The patient will get less ventilation, but if it means they will tolerate NIV better then you may accept this
- If air is leaking from the mouth with a nasal mask, use a chin strap or change to a mask which covers the mouth
- Check that the patient has their dentures in

Key Point | Terminology | **Practical Tip** | Physiology | How to do it

The lower straps on an NIV interface usually need to be much tighter than the upper straps.

Infection control

In acute respiratory failure, masks should be used on one patient and then discarded. For longer-term use at home, masks will last about six months if cared for well. They should be dismantled and washed in warm soapy water daily.

Key Point	Terminology	Practical Tip	Physiology	How to do it

For long-term use at home, NIV masks and circuits that look clean are unlikely to be a source of infection.

Nasal pillows

Nasal pillows, or cushions, consist of soft pads that fit just inside the patient's nostrils. They are less claustrophobic than a mask, and it is often easier to set them up without putting any pressure on the nasal bridge. The only down side is that they can be prone to displacement if the patient is moving around a lot. Many patients like to use nasal pillows for daytime NIV, because they can see better than with a mask and can wear their glasses. Even better in this regard are the large nasal cannulae designed for NIV, with soft ends which fit tightly inside the nostrils.

Mouthpieces

You can also use a mouthpiece for patients who need to use NIV during the daytime, for example patients with neuromuscular diseases. This could be a simple mouthpiece such as that sometimes used with a nebuliser, if the patient needs only a few breaths of NIV now and then. A flanged mouthpiece may be better if NIV is needed for slightly longer periods. It is possible to use a mouthpiece for overnight NIV — some patients with neuromuscular disorders affecting their arms or hands may find it easier to set themselves up on NIV if they use a mouthpiece rather than a mask (see Chapter 9).

Full-face masks

Full-face masks cover the nose and mouth, but also extend up over the eyes. Some patients find them very comfortable. They seem to work well in palliative care, perhaps because the masks don't get in the way of vision so much. The dead-space is greater, and the size of the mask can dampen the swings in pressure and hence render ventilation less effective. They can be used as a temporary measure to relieve pressure areas.

Key Point | Terminology | Practical Tip | Physiology | How to do it

Larger masks tend to increase dead-space.

Key Point | Terminology | Practical Tip | **Physiology** | How to do it

Equipment dead-space

We've already mentioned the problem of re-breathing, when we looked at how to connect a ventilator to the mask. If we allow our patient to breathe out into the tubing, they will then breathe in the air they have just exhaled. The whole circuit would be called "dead-space". We overcome this by putting an exhalation valve or port into the circuit. There is still a small amount of dead-space between the patient and the expiratory port (Figure 5.1). If you want to quantify this, for example in an experimental study, fill that part of the circuit up with water and pour it into a measuring jug.

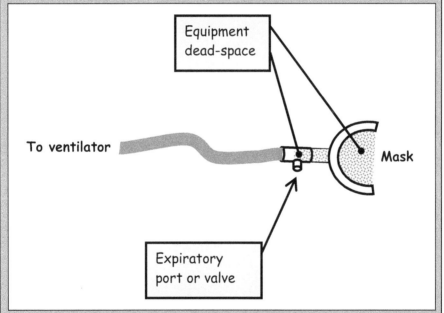

Figure 5.1 Equipment dead-space, from which exhaled air will be re-breathed on the next breath in.

Hybrid masks

Hybrid masks are oro-nasal masks, but with nasal pillows inside them. They are worth a try if you can't get a good seal with a nasal or oro-nasal mask, or if the patient is developing nasal bridge pressure sores.

Helmets

Helmets which fit right over the patient's head can sometimes be useful in acute respiratory failure. Breathless patients may tolerate them better than a mask. They work reasonably well with CPAP, but the large volume and general "springiness" of this system tend to dampen out the pressure swings during NIV. Smaller pressure swings means less ventilation.

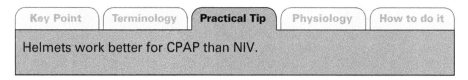

Key Point	Terminology	**Practical Tip**	Physiology	How to do it

Helmets work better for CPAP than NIV.

What should you keep in stock?

If you are starting an acute NIV service, see if there are any anaesthetic face masks already in use on your unit which are being used for CPAP. If they are any good, stick with these but make sure you have at least three different sizes in two different styles. If you are already using nasal masks to treat obstructive sleep apnoea, it probably makes sense to stick with the same style — make sure you have at least five different sizes, including some very small ones. My next choice would be a few sets of nasal pillows, to get you out of trouble if pressure over the bridge of the nose starts to damage the skin. Most units have a variety of different makes of face and nasal masks in stock. Different patients find different styles more comfortable. If you can't get a good fit with the first two or three you try then you are likely to end up trying every mask you have.

Key Point | Terminology | Practical Tip | Physiology | **How to do it**

Prevent nasal bridge pressure sores
- Choose the mask carefully
- Don't over-tighten the straps
- At the first sign of redness:
    - Put a protective dressing on the nose
    - Try a very small mask that just fits over the tip of the nose
    - Try an oro-nasal mask which takes most of the pressure on the forehead
    - Try nasal pillows
    - Try a full-face mask
    - Use different styles of mask for day and night

Summary

- Use an oro-nasal mask first in acute respiratory failure
- Use a nasal mask first in chronic respiratory failure (except in motor neurone disease, where oro-nasal is a better first bet)
- You'll need to keep quite a wide selection in stock
- Nasal pillows, full-face masks, mouthpieces and helmets are alternatives to masks, which are sometimes useful

6
Respiratory Failure

Learning points

By the end of this chapter you should be able to:

- **Distinguish between type 1 and type 2 respiratory failure**
- **List three reasons why a patient might develop type 2 respiratory failure**
- **Work out from some blood gas results whether type 2 respiratory failure is acute or chronic**
- **Explain why NIV tends to work best in type 2 respiratory failure**
- **Define FiO$_2$**

Let's think in a little more detail about respiratory failure. Most of the evidence for the effectiveness of NIV is in patients with type 2 respiratory failure. What does "type 2" mean?

Type 1 and type 2 respiratory failure

In type 2 respiratory failure there isn't enough air getting to the gas-exchanging part of the lungs. Carbon dioxide isn't removed effectively, so the PaCO$_2$ rises. We've already noted that this is called hypercapnia.

Key Point	Terminology	Practical Tip	Physiology	How to do it

In type 2 respiratory failure the $PaCO_2$ is elevated.

In type 2 respiratory failure the PaO_2 will be low, unless the patient is breathing supplementary oxygen, but the main issue is failure of ventilation rather than oxygenation.

Key Point	Terminology	Practical Tip	Physiology	How to do it

Inspired oxygen concentration
You will come across the term FiO_2. This means the fraction of the inspired gas that is oxygen. As you know, about 21% of air is oxygen, so the FiO_2 would be 0.21. A patient breathing 60% oxygen has an FiO_2 of 0.60. Sometimes FiO_2 is written as a percentage (e.g. FiO_2=60%), which is a bit confusing.

Causes of type 2 (hypercapnic) respiratory failure

Type 2 respiratory failure develops in three main situations:

- The *work* asked of the respiratory muscles is too great for them to sustain. Our patient with scoliosis had a deformed ribcage, the stiffness of which made it difficult for the respiratory muscles to expand
- The respiratory *muscles* are weak, and unable to ventilate the lungs. This is what happens in muscular dystrophy
- Central respiratory *drive* is impaired, and the respiratory muscles aren't told to ventilate the lungs. Poor central drive is seen with some diseases of the central nervous system and in the obesity-hypoventilation syndrome

I like the analogy which is sometimes used of a person who has to carry a box across a room. They might fail because the box is too heavy, because they are weak, or because their motivation (or drive) to do the task is not high.

Work, muscles and drive may all play a part in the same patient. In COPD, lots of ventilation is wasted moving air through parts of the lung that don't exchange gas well (dead-space), so the **work** of breathing is high; the inspiratory **muscles** don't work very effectively because the chest is at such a high lung volume (try breathing for a minute or so with a normal tidal volume, but up near total lung capacity — it's hard work); and many COPD patients have poor respiratory **drive** (they are sometimes called "blue bloaters" because they are cyanosed, overweight and oedematous).

| Key Point | Terminology | Practical Tip | **Physiology** | How to do it |

Alveolar ventilation and dead-space
Total ventilation is the amount of air going in and out of the lungs. You calculate this by multiplying the breathing rate by the size of each breath (Vt). The result is expressed in litres per minute.

Some of this ventilation is "wasted" on dead-space. Dead-space has three components:

• In NIV, equipment dead-space (which we discussed in Chapter 5)
• Parts of the lung which do not have alveoli, such as the trachea and bronchi
• Parts which do have alveoli but do not exchange gas with the blood particularly well

The bit without alveoli is called "anatomical" dead-space (Figure 6.1), but we are much more interested in the total amount of wasted ventilation — called "physiological" dead-space (Figure 6.2).

cont ...

Key Point   Terminology   Practical Tip   **Physiology**   How to do it

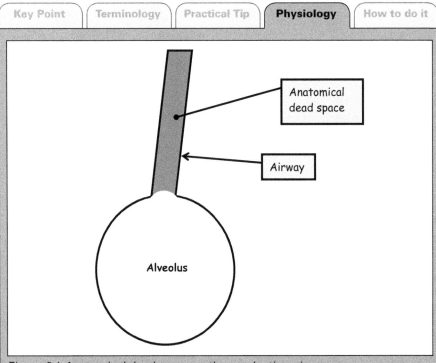

Figure 6.1 Anatomical dead-space — the conducting airways.

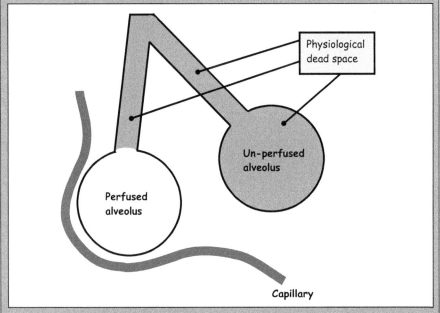

Figure 6.2 Physiological dead-space, which includes under-perfused alveoli.

cont ...

| Key Point | Terminology | Practical Tip | **Physiology** | How to do it |

The amount of ventilation getting to the gas-exchanging part of the lungs is called "alveolar ventilation" and is calculated as follows:

Breathing rate x (tidal volume – physiological dead-space)

Physiological dead-space in normal lungs is around one-third of tidal volume.

Acute or chronic?

The next thing we need to decide is whether the patient has acute or chronic hypercapnia. This is quite important in COPD, because NIV works best when the $PaCO_2$ has gone up during an acute illness or exacerbation.

CO_2 in the blood combines with water (H_2O) to create carbonic acid (H_2CO_3), which dissociates into bicarbonate ions (HCO_3^-) and hydrogen ions (H^+):

$$CO_2 + H_2O = H_2CO_3 = H^+ + HCO_3^-$$

H^+ is an acid. This is a "respiratory" acidosis because the cause is CO_2, as opposed to a "metabolic" acidosis where the acid comes from somewhere else (ketones or lactate for example). Acidosis is a low pH level — less than 7.35 — or a high hydrogen ion concentration (see appendix 4 for conversion table).

| Key Point | Terminology | **Practical Tip** | Physiology | How to do it |

Watch out for lactic acidosis caused by too much nebulised salbutamol in a patient admitted with an acute exacerbation of COPD. Also, make sure that patients with diabetes mellitus stop their metformin when they are ill. Both these drugs are infrequent but important causes of metabolic acidosis.

The pH level is related to the ratio of HCO_3^- (an alkali, sometimes also called a base) to CO_2. Normally these are exactly balanced (Figure 6.3).

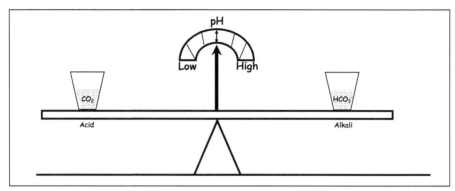

Figure 6.3 Normal pH is maintained by a balance between acid and alkali.

When the CO_2 goes up acutely, there is too much acid (the CO_2) — the scales tip over (Figure 6.4)

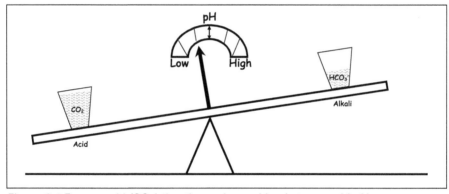

Figure 6.4 Excess acid (CO_2) tips the scales and leads to an acid pH.

The kidneys will try to get the pH back to normal by increasing the concentration of bicarbonate (Figure 6.5).

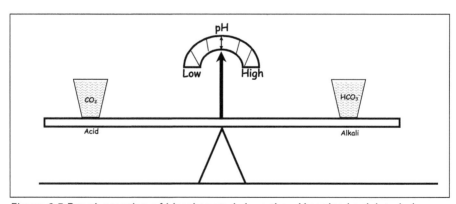

Figure 6.5 Renal retention of bicarbonate brings the pH scales back into balance.

This compensatory mechanism is of more relevance in some diseases than others. For example, you will probably want to consider NIV in a patient with scoliosis, obesity or muscular dystrophy who is hypercapnic, irrespective of the pH level. In COPD, NIV works mainly in acute hypercapnic respiratory failure, when the pH level will be low.

Key Point	Terminology	Practical Tip	Physiology	How to do it

In respiratory acidosis, the $PaCO_2$ is greater than 6 kPa and the pH level is less than 7.35. If the bicarbonate is greater than 30 mmol/l then the $PaCO_2$ has been high for some time — probably several days or more.

Key Point	Terminology	Practical Tip	**Physiology**	How to do it

Acid base diagrams
You'll probably have come across acid-base diagrams. They can be a bit intimidating when all the possible acid-base disturbances have been included. Let's start with a case of acute respiratory acidosis, where a high $PaCO_2$ leads to a low pH (Figure 6.6). The arrow travels along a line dictated by the bicarbonate concentration, which is normal at 25 mmol/l in this example.

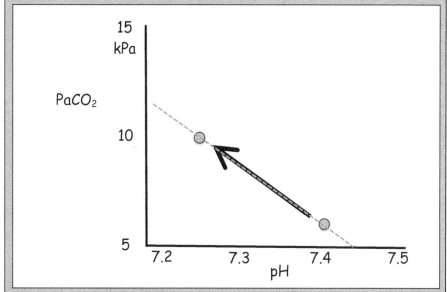

Figure 6.6 Fall in pH in an acute respiratory acidosis.

cont ...

Key Point | Terminology | Practical Tip | **Physiology** | How to do it

Retention of bicarbonate by the kidneys creates a new bicarbonate line on the diagram, with the pH returning to the normal range despite $PaCO_2$ remaining elevated (Figure 6.7).

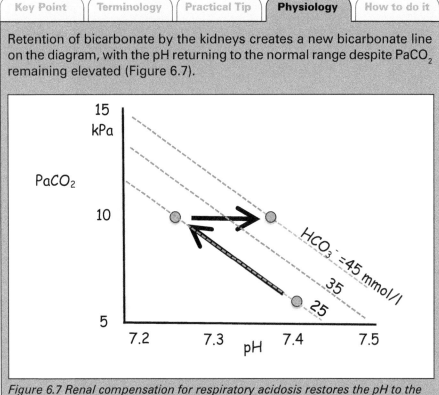

Figure 6.7 Renal compensation for respiratory acidosis restores the pH to the normal range.

Type 1 respiratory failure

In type 1 respiratory failure, there is plenty of air getting into the lungs, but they are not very effective at getting oxygen from the air across into the bloodstream. The PaO_2 is therefore low. Carbon dioxide is much more soluble than oxygen, which makes it much easier to wash out than it is to get oxygen in, so in type 1 respiratory failure the $PaCO_2$ is normal — it may even be low if the patient hyperventilates in an attempt to get more oxygen in.

Key Point | Terminology | Practical Tip | Physiology | How to do it

Type 2 respiratory failure is a failure of ventilation, hence non-invasive ventilation tends to work well. Type 1 respiratory failure is a failure of oxygenation rather than ventilation, therefore NIV is less effective.

The physiology of hypoxia is quite complex, but the most important process is the mismatching of ventilation and perfusion. For the moment it is sufficient to say that type 1 respiratory failure is failure of oxygenation and indicates lung disease. The more severe the hypoxia, the less likely the patient is to benefit from NIV (which is also true in type 2 respiratory failure).

| Key Point | Terminology | Practical Tip | Physiology | **How to do it** |

Diagnose respiratory failure from arterial blood gases
- Check what FiO_2 the patient was breathing when the sample was taken
- Is the PaO_2 is too low?
- This depends on age and FiO_2, as we'll see later
- Is the $PaCO_2$ >6 kPa?
- If it is, then this is type 2 respiratory failure
- Is the pH level less than 7.35?
- If the $PaCO_2$ is high and the pH level is low, this is an acute respiratory acidosis
- Is the HCO_3^- >30 mmol/l?
- If it is, this is a chronic respiratory acidosis
- Ignore all the other bits of data that are invariably printed out on the report — they don't add anything to the diagnosis of respiratory failure

| **Key Point** | Terminology | Practical Tip | Physiology | How to do it |

Hypoxia is much more dangerous than hypercapnia.

Summary

- Type 2 respiratory failure is an elevated $PaCO_2$
- A low pH level indicates that the high $PaCO_2$ is an acute problem that the kidneys have not yet had time to compensate for
- NIV works best in type 2 respiratory failure
- In both type 1 and type 2 respiratory failure, the more hypoxic the patient is, the less likely they are to benefit from NIV

7
Motor Neurone Disease

Learning points

By the end of this chapter you should be able to:

- List the symptoms and signs that suggest a patient with motor neurone disease has critical respiratory muscle weakness
- Describe how bulbar involvement impacts on the effectiveness of NIV

NIV helps some patients with motor neurone disease (MND), particularly those without bulbar involvement, relieving symptoms and prolonging life. Others find it less beneficial and there is a danger that struggling to get used to NIV can become one more thing to add to their burden. In this chapter we'll look at some general principles which will help you decide when to consider NIV in MND, but these are often difficult decisions for which you really only get a feel when you've been working with this group of patients for a while.

Key Point	Terminology	Practical Tip	Physiology	How to do it

In MND, NIV works best for patients with symptomatic diaphragm weakness but well-preserved bulbar function.

Respiratory muscle weakness

Some patients just have diaphragm paralysis when they first present with MND. This group tend to do really well on NIV, which helps them lie flat in bed and get a good night's sleep. The diagnosis of MND may only become apparent at a later date when they develop limb or bulbar signs.

Key Point	Terminology	**Practical Tip**	Physiology	How to do it

Keep checking for fasciculation in the limb muscles of patients who present with isolated diaphragm paralysis, in case the underlying diagnosis is MND.

Intercostal muscle paralysis may not be noticed by patients with MND if their diaphragm is still working, particularly when their mobility is already limited by limb muscle weakness. You should be able to spot this by the lack of ribcage expansion when you ask them to take a deep breath in. Measurement of VC will give you a more objective assessment. As with other muscle diseases, respiratory failure is unlikely if the VC is above 1.5 litres. (Supine VC is better than sitting in this regard, but many patients find it difficult to get on and off a couch.) Watch out for patients whose VC falls by more than 500mls between clinic visits — usually every 2-3 months in MND — and consider a trial of NIV before they get into trouble.

Key Point	Terminology	**Practical Tip**	Physiology	How to do it

Respiratory failure is unlikely in MND if the VC is greater than 1.5 litres.

Key Point	Terminology	Practical Tip	Physiology	**How to do it**

Diagnose bilateral diaphragm paralysis

- Ask the patient what happens to their breathing when they lie down. Normally, you increase the tone in your diaphragm when you lie down — if a patient is unable to do this, the contents of their abdomen push up into their ribcage and make them breathless; (the same thing happens when they walk into a swimming pool)
- Ask them if they sleep propped up in bed; patients with bilateral diaphragm paralysis sleep with lots of pillows, or in a chair

cont ...

Key Point | Terminology | Practical Tip | Physiology | **How to do it**

- Put your hand on the patient's epigastric region during quiet tidal breathing whilst they are sitting down. Keep your hand there and ask them a question or two. Normally, the ribcage and abdomen move outwards during inspiration (Figure 7.1). If the diaphragm is paralysed, you may be able to see or feel paradoxical abdominal motion (inward motion during inspiration) when they take a slightly deeper breath in before speaking (Figure 7.2)
- Ask them to sniff, whilst you feel for paradoxical abdominal motion
- If you're not sure about the presence of paradox, lie them down and do the same things
- If you're still not sure, ask them to see if they can push your hand upwards with their abdominal wall when they sniff; (normal contraction of the diaphragm pushes the abdominal contents down which pushes the anterior abdominal wall outwards)
- Measure VC seated and lying. If the lying value is more than 15% lower, then this is a pointer to diaphragm paralysis
- Measure maximum inspiratory (MIP) and expiratory (MEP) mouth pressures. In isolated diaphragm paralysis, MIP is low but MEP is normal; (if MEP is also reduced, this indicates expiratory muscle involvement)
- If you are still in doubt, measure oesophageal and gastric pressures, using pressure transducers or balloons

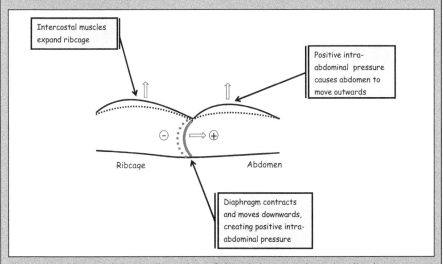

Intercostal muscles expand ribcage

Positive intra-abdominal pressure causes abdomen to move outwards

Ribcage   Abdomen

Diaphragm contracts and moves downwards, creating positive intra-abdominal pressure

Figure 7.1 Normal (outward) motion of the abdomen when the diaphragm contracts during inspiration. The ribcage also moves outwards, despite the negative intra-thoracic pressure, because of the action of the external intercostal muscles.

cont ...

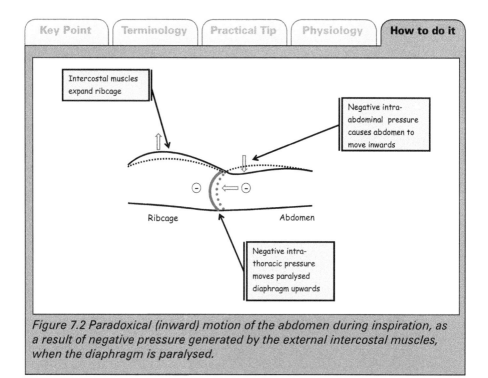

Figure 7.2 Paradoxical (inward) motion of the abdomen during inspiration, as a result of negative pressure generated by the external intercostal muscles, when the diaphragm is paralysed.

If the intercostal muscles as well as the diaphragm are weak, the patient will resort to the accessory neck muscles. These are small muscles which are a last resort in terms of breathing. They only produce a small tidal volume, so the patient will probably speed up their respiratory rate in order to achieve an adequate minute ventilation. It's time to start NIV.

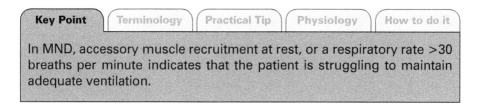

In MND, accessory muscle recruitment at rest, or a respiratory rate >30 breaths per minute indicates that the patient is struggling to maintain adequate ventilation.

If the $PaCO_2$ rises above 6 kPa then this is crisis point. This only happens when there is severe respiratory muscle weakness (Figure 7.3). Don't wait until the next day. Get on and try NIV.

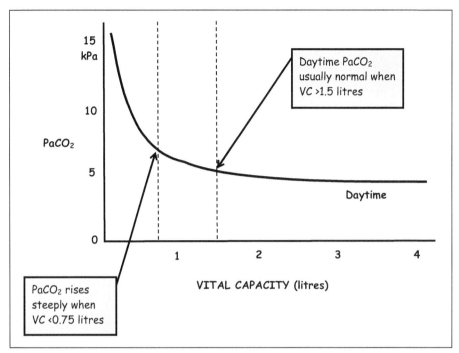

Figure 7.3 PaCO$_2$ starts to rise once the vital capacity is below 1.5 litres. It rises more steeply below 0.75 litres.

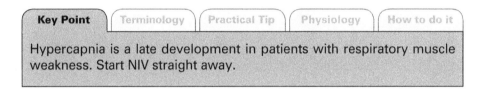

Key Point | Terminology | Practical Tip | Physiology | How to do it

Hypercapnia is a late development in patients with respiratory muscle weakness. Start NIV straight away.

Bulbar involvement and respiratory tests

Clinical assessment of respiratory muscle function is particularly important in MND patients with bulbar involvement. They often struggle with spirometry, even if you use a mask rather than a mouthpiece. If their VC is greater than 1.5 litres then they are likely to be fine from the respiratory point of view, since their true VC is at least 1.5 litres and may be considerably higher. If the VC is low, you need to try and work out if this really reflects respiratory muscle weakness, or whether they just have a problem performing spirometry. Other tests have been tried, such as sniff inspiratory pressure (SNIP), but they have all been disappointing. The best thing to do is just watch the patient breathing quietly at rest, looking at rate, chest and abdominal expansion and accessory recruitment. Then ask them to take a deep breath in and see what they can do. Your own VC will be up to ten times greater than your tidal volume, and you should be able to see whether your patient with MND has a similar pattern. If tidal volume and VC look pretty much the same, then there isn't a great deal of reserve and it may be time to start thinking about potential respiratory issues.

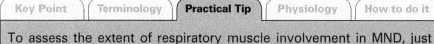

| Key Point | Terminology | **Practical Tip** | Physiology | How to do it |

To assess the extent of respiratory muscle involvement in MND, just watch the patient breathing quietly. Then ask them to take a deep breath in. With experience, you will be able to spot those patients who are running into trouble, even if they can't do breathing tests.

Sleep disturbance

Waking at night is quite common in MND. This may be for a variety of reasons, of which hypoventilation during rapid eye movement (REM) sleep is the most relevant in terms of NIV. We've already seen in scoliosis how this is a particularly bad phase of sleep for respiratory patients. If you were to measure $PaCO_2$ (or estimate it using a transcutaneous CO_2 monitor) during sleep in patients with muscle disease, you would find that it was higher than the daytime level during non-REM sleep, and higher still during REM sleep (Figure 7.4).

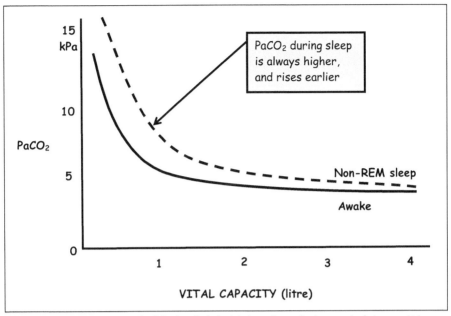

Figure 7.4 During sleep, PaCO$_2$ is slightly higher than during wakefulness. It is higher still in REM sleep.

Have a low threshold for requesting overnight oximetry, which is simple and easy to perform. Bear in mind, however, that just because the oxygen saturation drops this doesn't necessarily mean that the patient needs treatment — there need to be some symptoms of sleep disturbance, or daytime sleepiness, which have the potential to be improved by NIV. Also, keep an eye out for the occasional patient with obstructive sleep apnoea secondary to bulbar muscle weakness.

Ventilator settings

Use pressure-control, not pressure-support, since your aim is to rest the respiratory muscles and provide effective ventilation. If you can, use an exhalation valve in the circuit. That way you get as much ventilation as possible for any given IPAP. (We'll come back to this in the next chapter.)

Pressure-support is an alternative mode if the aim of NIV is to relieve breathlessness and the patient is unable to relax onto pressure-control, accepting that you may not be correcting hypoventilation completely.

Interfaces

Oro-nasal masks are a good option to start with. MND patients may need more than one type of interface — nasal pillows for daytime, nose or oro-nasal mask at night, full-face mask if nasal soreness develops etc. — and their needs will change as their disease progresses.

Bulbar involvement and NIV

Patients with severe bulbar weakness generally don't get on very well with NIV. Some, however, do benefit from it. The only way to find this out is for them to try. Good secretion management is important beforehand. Set clear goals: these might be, for example, better sleep, more alert during the day, less breathless etc. If they are not achieved pretty early on, it will usually be better to abandon NIV and try alternatives.

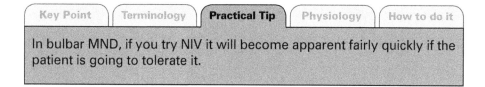

| Key Point | Terminology | **Practical Tip** | Physiology | How to do it |

In bulbar MND, if you try NIV it will become apparent fairly quickly if the patient is going to tolerate it.

Ventilator dependence

It is not uncommon in MND for your patient to progress from night-time NIV to complete ventilator dependence. Don't forget to put safety mechanisms in place when this happens: internal ventilator battery, spare ventilator, self-inflating bag etc. (See Chapter 45.)

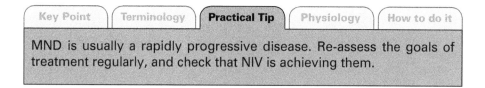

| Key Point | Terminology | **Practical Tip** | Physiology | How to do it |

MND is usually a rapidly progressive disease. Re-assess the goals of treatment regularly, and check that NIV is achieving them.

Cough

As we'll see later on, cough requires good inspiratory muscles to get air into the lungs, good laryngeal muscles to close the larynx whilst the expiratory muscles build up some pressure, and good expiratory muscle strength for the expulsive phase. Any or all of these may be abnormal in MND. Ask the patient to cough into a peak flow meter — they should be able to get 300 l/min or more. Less than 150 l/min and there is likely to be a problem expectorating secretions. If this is the case, the options to help cough are manually-assisted coughing, breath-stacking or a cough-assist device (Chapter 43).

Key Point	Terminology	**Practical Tip**	Physiology	How to do it

Every time a patient with MND attends clinic, check their VC, oxygen saturation and peak cough flow.

Key Point	Terminology	Practical Tip	**Physiology**	How to do it

Breath-stacking
This refers to the practice of stacking a few inspiratory breaths, with no exhalation in between. It is most commonly employed with a self-inflating "resuscitation" bag. A series of breaths are delivered to the patient, without them breathing out in-between. They close their glottis to hold the air in, then cough. This will, hopefully, be much stronger than after a single breath in.

There are two ways of stacking the inspired volume. The patient can close their glottis, and wait for you to deliver the next breath, or you can use a one-way valve in the circuit (Figure 7.5). The latter technique allows you to deliver quite a number of small breaths pretty quickly, and requires less co-ordination with the patient.

cont ...

Key Point | Terminology | Practical Tip | **Physiology** | How to do it

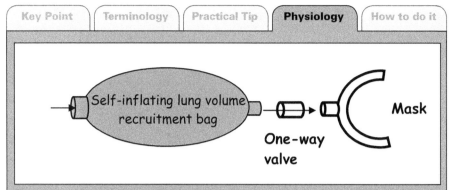

Figure 7.5 Circuit for breath-stacking, using a lung-volume recruitment bag.

Going back to our pressure-volume curve, you can see that with each stacked breath we will need to use a higher inflation pressure (Figure 7.6). Because the pressure source is us squeezing a bag, we don't refer to it as IPAP, but the principle is the same.

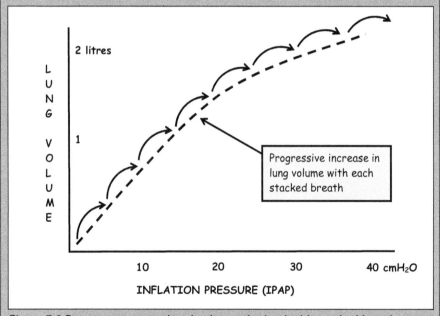

Figure 7.6 Pressure generated and volume obtained with stacked breaths.

If you just use the same pressure, you don't move any higher up the pressure-volume curve. That means no more air into the lungs. Using an NIV ventilator with the same target pressure for each breath is not breath-stacking.

cont ...

| Key Point | Terminology | Practical Tip | **Physiology** | How to do it |

If you have ever used a self-inflating resuscitation bag, you'll know that you don't really have any idea how much pressure you are generating. You just watch the chest to see that you are expanding it adequately. If you attach a pressure monitor during breath-stacking, you'll be surprised just how high it gets — 60 or 70 cmH$_2$O.

Volume-targeted ventilators (Chapter 40) are well-suited to breath-stacking. They push a fixed volume of air into the lungs, using whatever pressure it takes.

| **Key Point** | Terminology | Practical Tip | Physiology | How to do it |

A pressure-targeted ventilator cannot deliver stacked breaths, unless you push up the IPAP.

| Key Point | **Terminology** | Practical Tip | Physiology | How to do it |

Insufflation capacity
Insufflation capacity is the total volume exhaled after breath-stacking — a large volume implies good vocal cord function and is associated with the ability to expectorate secretions from the lungs.

The end of life

At some stage you'll need to have a discussion about withdrawal of NIV at the end of life. We'll look at all the issues in more detail in the chapter on Palliative Care (Chapter 29). Difficult decisions are surprisingly uncommon in MND. Most patients reach a stage where they have just had enough. They stop using NIV quite so much and slowly decline. Breathlessness may be less of an issue than you might expect. This is because the patient is no longer fighting to maintain a normal PaCO$_2$. As they become more drowsy, they will reach for NIV less. Strive to maintain their dignity. Respect their wishes, currently or previously expressed. The family will need your support.

Summary

- NIV helps many, but not all, patients with MND
- NIV works best for those with diaphragm paralysis without much bulbar involvement
- Watch out for accessory muscle recruitment at rest indicating that the patient is struggling to maintain adequate ventilation
- Hypercapnia is a late development in those with respiratory muscle weakness and indicates the need to start NIV

8
Pressure-Support and Pressure-Control

Learning points

By the end of this chapter you should be able to:

- **Define pressure-control ventilation**
- **Define pressure-support ventilation**
- **Describe how expiratory positive airway pressure can be added to produce bi-level NIV**

There are lots of different modes of ventilation. As we have mentioned already, you only really need to know in detail about two: pressure-support and pressure-control.

Pressure-control ventilation

We noted when we started our patient with scoliosis on NIV, pressure-control is the mode used by many patients on long-term ventilation at home. It is also sometimes needed for acute respiratory failure, for example if pressure-support fails or in patients with ventilatory pump problems (drive, muscle or chest wall problems). At the risk of labouring the point, and perhaps of over-simplification, you could think of pressure-control as **delivering** ventilation rather than just providing a bit of support.

Just to re-cap, the features of pressure-control are as follows:

- **It is a pressure-targeted mode — the ventilator is set to deliver the same pressure with each breath**
- **The duration of inspiration is determined ("controlled") by the ventilator**
- **The respiratory rate is also determined by the ventilator. This is not just a back-up rate: the patient will be ventilated at this rate most of the time**
- **The patient can trigger a breath, but they usually don't. If they do, it will be the same duration as an un-triggered breath**

We've already alluded to the use of pressure-control NIV with an exhalation valve. For the purposes of this book, I am going to call this mode "IPPV", which stands for intermittent positive pressure ventilation (Figure 8.1). This is to distinguish it from bi-level pressure-control, which we'll talk about in a moment.

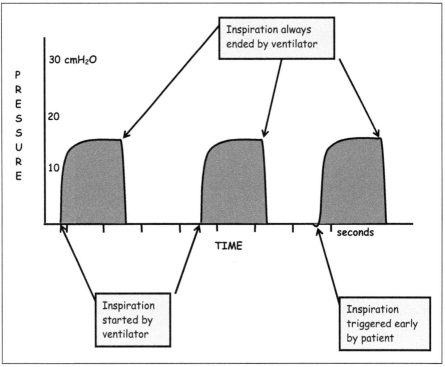

Figure 8.1 Intermittent positive pressure ventilation (IPPV). This is IPAP with no expiratory pressure, and it requires a circuit with an expiratory valve.

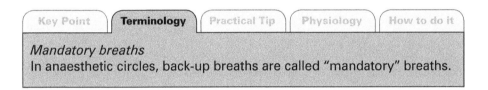

In this book, "IPPV" means pressure-control NIV with an exhalation valve in the circuit and no EPAP.

Pressure-support ventilation

In pressure-support ventilation, the only thing we set is the level of pressure that the ventilator will deliver with each breath. The timing is determined by the patient, who triggers the beginning and end of each breath (Figure 8.2). Pressure-support is so-called because the patient is breathing spontaneously with their own breathing rhythm, but with each breath they are being helped (supported) to breathe in by the IPAP from the ventilator. In an acute situation, the patient's breathing rate and pattern are liable to change as they get better. The beauty of pressure-support is that the ventilator will follow any changes, without you having to continually adjust the rate and inspiratory:expiratory (I:E) ratio. There is always a back-up setting if the patient's breathing becomes too slow, and you do have to set the rate and I:E ratio for that — we'll come back to this later.

Mandatory breaths
In anaesthetic circles, back-up breaths are called "mandatory" breaths.

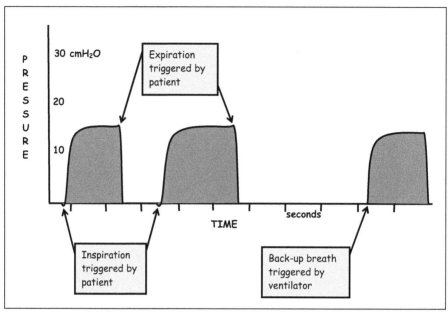

Figure 8.2 Pressure-time trace of three breaths during pressure-support ventilation. The patient triggers each breath, so the interval between breaths is variable. The target pressure of 15 cmH₂O is the same for each breath, but they are of different lengths, since the patient also triggers the switch across into expiration.

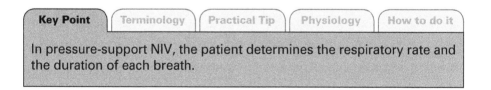

Key Point | Terminology | Practical Tip | Physiology | How to do it

In pressure-support NIV, the patient determines the respiratory rate and the duration of each breath.

Bi-level pressure-support

You will probably be familiar with the use of CPAP in ICU or HDU to keep the lungs fully expanded, for example in patients with pneumonia, and to provide a bit of extra pressure to help with the transfer of oxygen across into the bloodstream. CPAP involves application of the same pressure throughout the breathing cycle. It is also used in the treatment of obstructive sleep apnoea, to keep the upper airway open during sleep. As we noted in Chapter 2, the pressure-time trace during CPAP is a straight line (Figure 8.3).

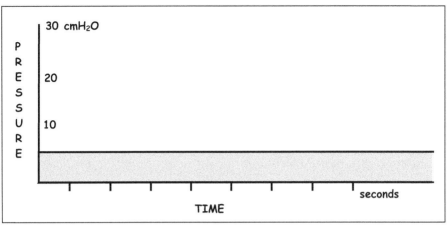

Figure 8.3 Pressure-time trace of CPAP at 5 cmH$_2$O.

If we combine pressure-support and CPAP, we get a high pressure during inspiration (IPAP) with a lower background pressure during expiration. The background pressure is no longer called CPAP (because it is not "continuous") but becomes EPAP — expiratory positive airway pressure. The combination of IPAP and EPAP is bi-level NIV (Figure 8.4).

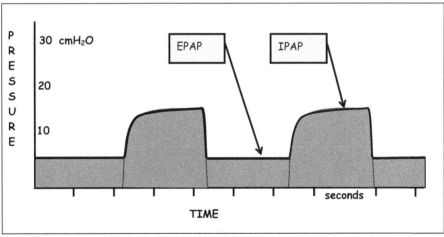

Figure 8.4 Pressure-time trace of two breaths during bi-level NIV, with an IPAP of 15 cmH$_2$O and an EPAP of 5 cmH$_2$O.

Pressure-support is almost always combined with EPAP. Bi-level pressure-support NIV is the main mode of NIV used for acute exacerbations of COPD. For many of you this will be the mode of NIV with which you are most familiar.

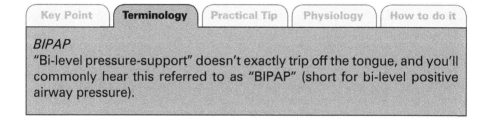

Key Point | Terminology | Practical Tip | Physiology | How to do it

Bi-level pressure-support is the most widely used mode for treating acute respiratory failure.

Adding EPAP has some physiological advantages, as we'll discuss later on. One useful effect of EPAP is that it allows us to use a very simple circuit — we'll see why in the next chapter.

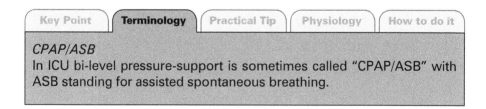

Key Point | **Terminology** | Practical Tip | Physiology | How to do it

BIPAP

"Bi-level pressure-support" doesn't exactly trip off the tongue, and you'll commonly hear this referred to as "BIPAP" (short for bi-level positive airway pressure).

Features of bi-level pressure-support NIV are:

- **It is a pressure-targeted mode of NIV, where we set the pressure that the ventilator reaches with each breath**
- **The patient determines the respiratory rate**
- **The patient determines the duration of inspiration and expiration, and hence the respiratory rate**
- **There is a back-up rate set on the ventilator**
- **Re-breathing is avoided by making a simple expiratory port in the mask or circuit**

Key Point | **Terminology** | Practical Tip | Physiology | How to do it

CPAP/ASB

In ICU bi-level pressure-support is sometimes called "CPAP/ASB" with ASB standing for assisted spontaneous breathing.

Bi-level pressure-control

Bi-level pressure-control also has IPAP and EPAP, with the features of a control mode we already looked at:

- The duration of inspiration is determined by the ventilator
- The respiratory rate is also determined by the ventilator. This is not just a back-up rate: the patient will be ventilated at this rate most of the time
- The patient can trigger a breath, but they usually don't. If they do, it will be the same duration as an un-triggered breath
- It utilises an expiratory port in a single-tube circuit, in the same way as bi-level pressure-support

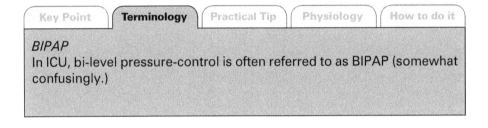

| Key Point | **Terminology** | Practical Tip | Physiology | How to do it |

BIPAP
In ICU, bi-level pressure-control is often referred to as BIPAP (somewhat confusingly.)

| Key Point | Terminology | Practical Tip | **Physiology** | How to do it |

Inspiratory and expiratory flow
We have looked at how the volume of the lung increases rapidly when we apply pressure during NIV, using the pressure-volume curve. We have seen how pressure goes up and down with time, so let's plot volume against time (Figure 8.5).

cont ...

Key Point   Terminology   Practical Tip   **Physiology**   How to do it

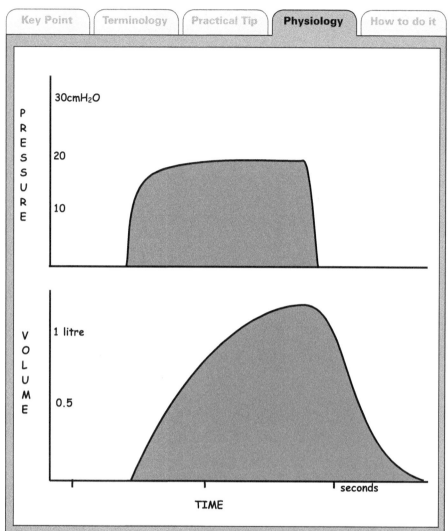

Figure 8.5 Pressure and volume plotted against time for a single breath of IPPV.

You'll notice that the volume change lags behind the pressure change — on our diagrams volume doesn't have the same square profile. This is because it takes a bit of time for the air to flow in, and there are "elastic" forces in the lungs and ribcage which resist deformation. We'll come back to this later.

cont ...

Key Point | Terminology | Practical Tip | **Physiology** | How to do it

The rate of change in volume is flow. If we plot volume and flow, you can see that inspiratory flow increases rapidly and then tails off, mirroring the slope of the volume trace (Figure 8.6).

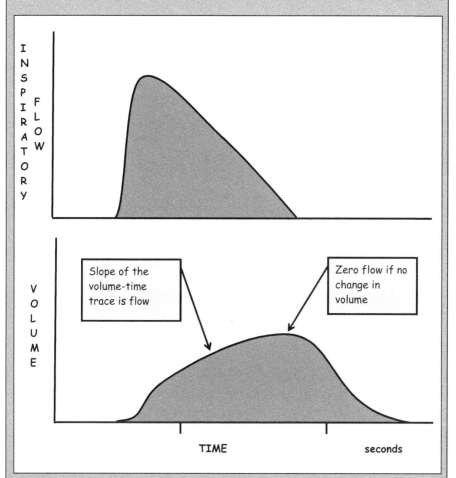

Figure 8.6 Rate of change in volume is flow. Flow tails off towards the end of inspiration, as the lung gets up to tidal volume.

Add expiratory flow (Figure 8.7), and we have the sort of plot you will see on ventilator displays.

cont ...

Key Point   Terminology   Practical Tip   **Physiology**   How to do it

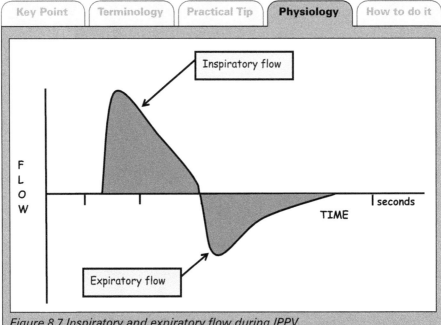

Figure 8.7 Inspiratory and expiratory flow during IPPV.

The inspiratory flow is produced by the positive pressure generated by our non-invasive ventilator. During inspiration, stretching of the elastic tissue of the lungs and ribcage stores potential energy in them. It is this energy which produces expiratory flow. If you need to, you can augment this by contracting your expiratory muscles.

Key Point   **Terminology**   Practical Tip   Physiology   How to do it

Ventilator cycling: time or flow?
In pressure-control, the beginning and end of each breath happens at a predetermined time. This is called time-cycling. In pressure-support, the beginning and end of each breath is determined by changes in flow, so this is a flow-cycled mode. Time-cycling may kick in if the patient's rate drops too low.

Summary

- Pressure-support provides a positive pressure in time with the patient's own breathing cycle to help them breathe in
- Bi-level pressure-support is pressure-support with expiratory pressure added
- The expiratory pressure is called EPAP
- Pressure-support is flow-cycled, pressure-control is time-cycled

9
Mouthpiece NIV

Learning points

By the end of this chapter you should be able to:

- **Give an example of when mouthpiece ventilation might be useful**
- **Set ventilator alarms so they don't go off during daytime mouthpiece ventilation**

When we talked about masks, it was obvious that these needed to be strapped into place. Somewhat surprisingly, some patients manage to keep a flanged mouthpiece in place at night, and prefer this to a mask. The main advantage is that there is nothing on the face to cause pressure sores. A good seal is possible, provided there isn't any weakness of the buccal muscles. Prolonged use of a mouthpiece can, however, cause distortion of the teeth.

A more common application of this technique is for top-up ventilation during the daytime. Most patients who use it have neuromuscular conditions causing severe respiratory muscle weakness. Think about mouthpiece NIV if your patient is almost ventilator-dependent, but can manage a few minutes of spontaneous breathing. It can help their independence, in that they can get onto NIV without having to get help to strap a mask in place. If they only need a few breaths (for example during meals, washing, shaving) it will be much more convenient than a mask.

The mouthpiece

For daytime mouthpiece NIV, use an unflanged mouthpiece (there may be some around somewhere in a cupboard of nebuliser equipment). With a bit of ingenuity, this can be mounted so that it is positioned just next to the patient. You could attach it to a wheelchair table with a semi-rigid mount, similar to a desktop lamp. Another alternative is a halter attached to the patient. Try a few different options so that they will be able just to turn their head and latch onto the mouthpiece. A few breaths of NIV, and they can resume their meal or conversation.

Ventilator settings

Originally mouthpiece ventilation used volume-targeted ventilators. It works just as well with modern pressure-targeted devices. Use pressure-control modes, and set the pressures, rate and I:E ratio at a level the patient finds comfortable.

Alarms

When a patient is awake and using a mouthpiece for top-up assisted breaths during the day, for example whilst eating or holding a conversation, they do not need an alarm to tell them that they have taken the mouthpiece out of their mouth. An alarm constantly going off is going to be an irritation. Some patients just keep their cheek up against the mouthpiece when they are not breathing through it, to keep the pressure above the alarm level. The mouthpiece causes a bit of resistance to flow, so there will usually be pressure within the circuit even when the patient is not connected. You can set the alarm below this level, but clearly it is important to increase the threshold again to detect disconnection during the night (Figure 9.1).

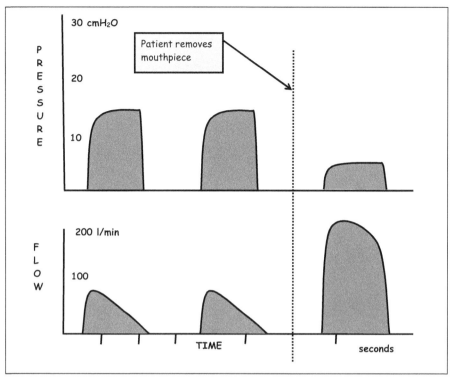

Figure 9.1 Pressure and flow during mouthpiece ventilation. When the patient is not attached to the mouthpiece, the ventilator pushes up the flow it delivers in an attempt to achieve the target pressure. You will need to adjust the low pressure or high-flow alarm for top-up assisted breaths during the daytime.

Key Point	Terminology	Practical Tip	**Physiology**	How to do it

Pressure, flow and resistance

You may have noticed in Figure 9.1 that there is still some IPAP even when the patient isn't connected to the ventilator. Why is this? Well, it depends where pressure is being measured.

Some ventilators will use an additional small-bore tube to measure pressure at the interface. This would be zero (or atmospheric) pressure in our example.

Most NIV ventilators measure pressure at the ventilator end of the circuit. There must be a pressure drop down the ventilator circuit in order to produce flow. Think of a garden hose: there is pressure at the tap, atmospheric pressure at the other end. If there wasn't any pressure from the mains water, no water would flow down the hose.

cont ...

The fall in pressure down a tube is called resistance. (The physical principles also apply to our bronchial tubes.) Resistance is proportional to the length of the tube; the longer the ventilator tubing, the greater the fall in pressure. Bear this in mind when you add extra bits of tubing, for example when you use a heated humidifier.

The tube diameter is particularly important, since resistance is inversely proportional to diameter to the power of 4. Halve the diameter of the tube and the resistance increases by a factor of 16 (2 x 2 x 2 x 2). It might be tempting to use a slightly smaller diameter tube, but even a small change in diameter has a considerable impact on the fall in pressure (resistance).

In a length of ventilator circuit tubing, the flow of air will be "laminar". This means it is smooth and free-flowing, rather like the water in the straight stretch of a river. If there are sharp bends, flow becomes "turbulent". (In our river, this would be seen as eddies round rocks or bridge piers.) Turbulent flow occurs when you add anything to the circuit tubing — angled connectors, humidifiers, filters, exhalation ports or valves, masks (Figure 9.2). It is particularly likely to happen when flow is very high, as it will be in our example when our patient removes the mouthpiece and the ventilator blows hard to try and achieve the target pressure.

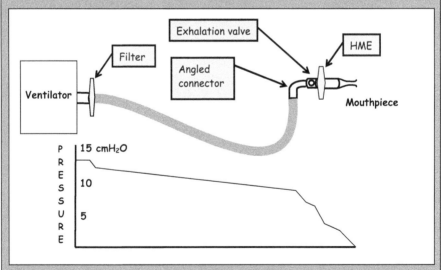

Figure 9.2 Fall in pressure down an NIV circuit, not connected to a patient, with high flow down the circuit. Any addition to the circuit will produce turbulent flow and a fall in pressure.

| Key Point | Terminology | **Practical Tip** | Physiology | How to do it |

Putting a heat-moisture exchanger in the circuit can be handy to provide added resistance, which prevents low-pressure or high-flow alarms going off as soon as the patient comes off the mouthpiece.

Summary

- Mouthpiece ventilation is a useful option for use during daytime in patients who are almost completely ventilator-dependent
- It requires a bit of ingenuity

10
Polio

Learning points

By the end of this chapter you should be able to:

- **Describe how polio can affect breathing**
- **List the key factors which predispose a patient with polio to develop hypercapnic respiratory failure**

The poliomyelitis virus infects lower motor neurones and prevents them from relaying signals from the central nervous system to the muscles. Before the introduction of vaccination, polio was a common cause of ventilatory failure. Much of what we know today about ventilation was learnt during polio epidemics. Some patients have been ventilated continuously at home since the 1950s.

From time to time you will probably come across patients with polio who slip into ventilatory failure many years after their original illness. The reasons for this late deterioration are not clear; it could be that the respiratory muscles which remain innervated are subject to normal ageing processes, having had years of coping with an increased load (for example, due to scoliosis).

Ventilatory failure as a late complication of polio

Features identifying the patients with polio who you need to keep under annual review in clinic are:

- **Previous need for artificial ventilation (such as an iron lung) during the acute illness**
- **Thoracic scoliosis, following paraspinal muscle paralysis**
- **A history of upper limb polio, which makes it much more likely that there was involvement of the respiratory muscles during the acute illness**
- **Vital capacity less than 50% predicted**
- **Obesity**

Key Point	Terminology	**Practical Tip**	Physiology	How to do it

See patients with polio who are at risk of respiratory failure, once a year in clinic. Ask about symptoms of nocturnal hypoventilation, frequency of chest infections etc. Look for right heart failure. Measure VC and check their arterial blood gases. Have a low threshold for doing overnight oximetry.

NIV in polio

NIV works well in polio. Initially nocturnal use will be enough, but sometimes a top-up in the middle of the day will become necessary. Use IPPV with an IPAP of 25-30 cmH$_2$O to start with. If you only have bi-level pressure-control, then keep the EPAP low.

Short or long-term NIV

Patients with polio experience a slow decline over several decades. As with any slowly progressive disease, the patient may not have been aware of this decline. Treatment of an acute episode of respiratory failure will improve their functional status, but generally to a level slightly below where they were (Figure 10.1).

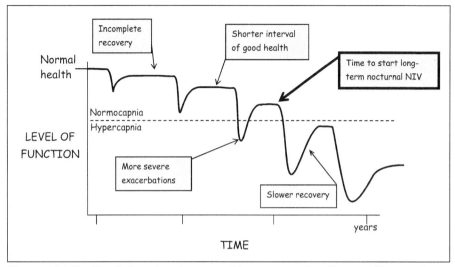

Figure 10.1 Decline in functional status with a progressive disease. After each acute illness, recovery is to a lower level than before that episode. The rate of decline tends to accelerate.

This pattern is seen in scoliosis, thoracoplasty and neuromuscular diseases. Perhaps surprisingly, it is also common in obesity. Do you really need to suggest long-term nocturnal NIV at the stage shown on Figure 10.1? The answer is yes, you probably do. Another acute episode is probably not that far away, then another. Any one of these might be life-threatening.

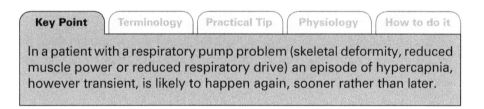

Key Point	Terminology	Practical Tip	Physiology	How to do it

In a patient with a respiratory pump problem (skeletal deformity, reduced muscle power or reduced respiratory drive) an episode of hypercapnia, however transient, is likely to happen again, sooner rather than later.

Supplementary oxygen

Don't rush to add in supplementary oxygen if the patient is sleeping better and their daytime arterial blood gases are improving. Add it in if, after a couple of months of nocturnal NIV, the mean peripheral oxygen saturation (SpO_2) overnight is less than 85%, particularly if there is clinical evidence of right heart failure.

Key Point	Terminology	**Practical Tip**	Physiology	How to do it

If you order oxygen for patients with chronic hypercapnic respiratory failure on NIV, tell the patient to use it only when they are on NIV at night and not during the day (when they are not using NIV). It is not like long-term oxygen therapy (LTOT) in COPD, which should be used for 12 or 15 hours per day. Supplementary oxygen without NIV can be dangerous in patients with chest wall problems, as in other causes of chronic type 2 respiratory failure, because it removes hypoxic drive.

Key Point	Terminology	Practical Tip	**Physiology**	How to do it

Improvement in daytime blood gases with nocturnal NIV
When you start a patient on NIV, their daytime arterial blood gases — both PaO_2 and $PaCO_2$ — tend to get steadily better over several months. Why?

• The breathing muscles could get stronger, because they get a rest at night (i.e. bigger capacity in our load/capacity/motivation model, Chapter 6)
• The lungs and/or ribcage could get easier to move (more compliant), because of the action of the ventilator at night (i.e. less load)
• Respiratory drive might pick up

The answer appears to be respiratory drive. Maximum mouth pressures, vital capacity etc., don't change much but respiratory drive picks up. The reasons for this are not clear, but correction of nocturnal hypoventilation is likely to be the most important factor.

Summary

• Some patients with polio slip into hypercapnic respiratory failure as a late complication
• NIV, usually just at night, works very well for them

11
Circuits

Learning points

By the end of this chapter you should be able to:

- Put together a circuit for bi-level pressure-support
- Describe why re-breathing would occur if the expiratory port were blocked
- Say why a bacterial filter should be placed over the ventilator outlet
- Demonstrate how you would set up this mode of ventilation for a patient with an acute exacerbation of COPD
- Put together a circuit for pressure-control using an exhalation valve
- Explain the consequences of failing to connect the exhalation valve to the circuit

A ventilator circuit needs to deliver air from the ventilator to the patient. We could do this by using a length of standard 22 mm tubing. The problem with a simple tube is that the patient breathes out into the tubing, and then breathes the same "stale" air back in again. You can try this for yourself just by breathing in and out of a length of tube — within a few breaths you start to feel pretty uncomfortable. This is because you are breathing back in air which you have breathed out, which is low in oxygen but high in CO_2 (Figure 11.1) This is called re-breathing, which would be inevitable if we just connected a patient to their ventilator with a length of tubing, as we saw in Chapter 2.

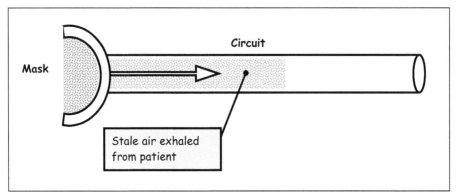

Figure 11.1 Exhaled air in the circuit tubing, which would be re-inhaled if there were no expiratory or exhalation valve.

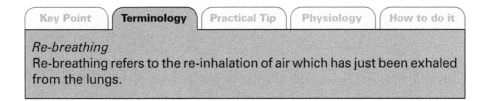

Key Point	**Terminology**	Practical Tip	Physiology	How to do it

Re-breathing
Re-breathing refers to the re-inhalation of air which has just been exhaled from the lungs.

The expiratory port

With bi-level NIV, the expiratory port is a small hole in the circuit, near to the mask. When the ventilator is pushing air into the patient, there is some leakage through this hole (Figure 11.2), but the ventilator is easily able to adjust for this.

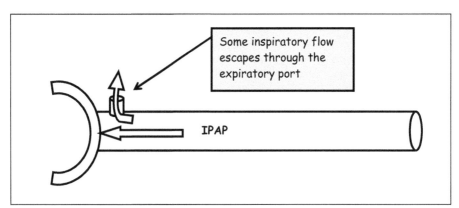

Some inspiratory flow escapes through the expiratory port

IPAP

Figure 11.2 During inspiration, there is some leakage of air out through the expiratory port.

When the patient breathes out, the hole isn't big enough for all the exhaled air to pass through — some of the exhaled air goes down the main tube (Figure 11.3).

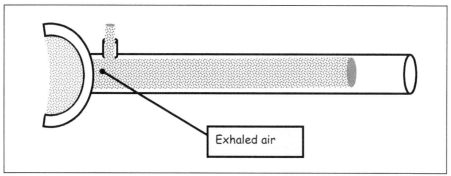

Figure 11.3 Exhaled air goes out of the expiratory port, and back down the ventilator tubing.

Later, as the flow from the patient tails off, the positive pressure in the circuit (EPAP) pushes the exhaled air back up the tube and out of the leakage hole (Figure 11.4).

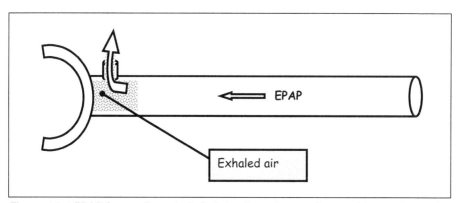

Figure 11.4 EPAP forces the exhaled air back up the ventilator tubing and out of the expiratory port. When IPAP comes along at the start of the next inspiration, there is no exhaled air left in the circuit.

Key Point	Terminology	Practical Tip	Physiology	How to do it

In bi-level ventilation there is a small hole, or exhalation port, in the circuit near the mask to vent out exhaled air.

There is nothing special about the hole in the tube. It needs to be about 5mm in diameter — too small and the flow isn't enough to blow out exhaled air. If it is too big, there will be so much flow that the ventilator may struggle to get enough pressure to the patient. Also, the ventilator may not be able to sense when the patient wants to breathe in.

Your circuits may already come with an expiratory port. These are deliberately designed to make them difficult to block off (or connect oxygen tubing to). However, it is not unheard of for someone who doesn't understand NIV to tape up the expiratory port, thinking it is a faulty circuit.

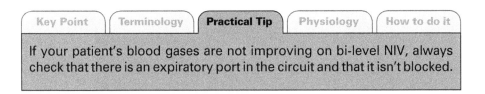

Key Point	Terminology	**Practical Tip**	Physiology	How to do it

If your patient's blood gases are not improving on bi-level NIV, always check that there is an expiratory port in the circuit and that it isn't blocked.

If the mask you are using has access ports on it, you can open these up as the exhalation ports. Some masks come with right-angle connectors which have perforations in to act as the expiratory port. Perforations built in to the top of the mask ought to be the best option for blowing out CO_2 with the least re-breathing (Figure 11.5).

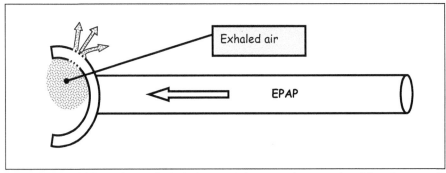

Exhaled air

EPAP

Figure 11.5 EPAP pushes exhaled air out of the vents in a mask, with only a small volume of equipment dead-space.

Start a patient on bi-level pressure-support
- Choose a mask, usually an oro-nasal mask
- Get the right straps to hold it in place
- Set up the circuit
- Turn the ventilator on
- If there is a choice of mode on the ventilator, choose bi-level pressure-support
- If the ventilator has an option with a back-up rate (e.g. assist/control) set it to 12 breaths per minute
- Set the IPAP to 12 cmH_2O
- Set the EPAP to 5 cmH_2O
- Hold the mask on the patient, and ask them to breathe in and out of the mask so they get used to the sensation of the pressure from the ventilator
- When they are settled, strap the mask in place
- Watch for a few minutes
- Check the oxygen saturation: if it is less than 88%, increase the IPAP to 20 cmH_2O. If this doesn't work, put an oxygen connector in the circuit and start 1 l/min of oxygen, or set the oxygen concentration on the ventilator to 28% if you have this facility*
- Set up appropriate monitoring*
- Write down the ventilator settings and oxygen flow rate
- Decide when you are going to re-evaluate (e.g. with a blood gas in one hour)*
- After discussion with all appropriate people, write down whether the patient is to be intubated if they deteriorate*

The steps marked * will make more sense in due course, but it will be easier to understand them if you have already done some basic NIV. If any of the steps <u>not</u> marked with a * are causing you concern, then go back a stage and re-read the relevant section.

Exhalation valves

Pressure-control ventilators designed for use at home may have an exhalation valve to prevent re-breathing, rather than the exhalation port we used for bi-level NIV (Figure 11.6). This exhalation valve is near the mask. It is closed when the ventilator is pushing air into the patient, so that the air doesn't escape through the valve rather than getting to the patient. It opens during expiration to let the air escape. (Very occasionally the diaphragm in the valve may split or become folded — you can dismantle the valve to check this, or just change the circuit.) You need an additional small tube to pressurise the valve to close it. I refer to this mode of NIV as IPPV.

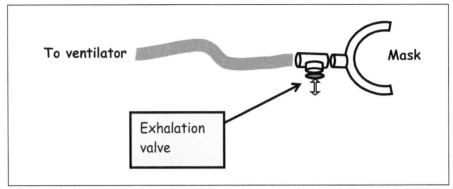

Figure 11.6 Exhalation valve between the circuit tubing and the mask

Key Point	Terminology	**Practical Tip**	Physiology	How to do it

If the small bore pressure-monitoring and exhalation-valve tubes have been connected the wrong way round, you will hear lots of air whooshing out of the expiratory valve during inspiration.

Key Point	Terminology	Practical Tip	Physiology	**How to do it**

Start a patient on IPPV
- Choose a mask, usually a nasal mask
- Get the right straps to hold it in place
- Set up the circuit
- Count the patient's spontaneous respiratory rate
- Turn the ventilator on
- Set the ventilator rate to the spontaneous rate
- Adjust the timing of the ventilator so that the inspiration and expiration are approximately the same as the patient's own spontaneous breaths
- Set the IPAP to 20 cmH$_2$O
- Hold the mask on the patient, and ask them to breathe in and out of the mask so they get used to the sensation of the pressure from the ventilator
- When they have grown accustomed to NIV, strap the mask in place
- Watch for a few minutes

cont ...

- Adjust the mask to minimise leaks
- Adjust the pressure up or down, within the range 15-30 cmH$_2$O, to the lowest level that gives good chest expansion
- See if the patient feels comfortable with a slightly slower respiratory rate
- Check the oxygen saturation: if it less than 88%, increase the IPAP. If this doesn't work, put an oxygen connector in the circuit and start 1 l/min of oxygen
- Write down the ventilator settings

If the exhalation port or valve is placed at the ventilator end of the circuit rather than the mask end, the patient will inevitably re-breathe only exhaled air (Figure 11.7). This is an easy mistake to make — always check the circuit.

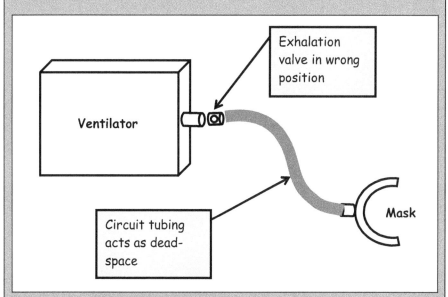

Figure 11.7 If the circuit is assembled with the exhalation port or valve at the wrong end, re-breathing is inevitable.

Infection control

In acute respiratory failure, circuits should be used on one patient only. There is no need to change the circuit daily — as with masks, circuits that look clean are generally fine from a microbiological point of view.

For long-term NIV at home, circuits should be washed once a week in warm soapy water — or in a dish washer — and hung up to dry thoroughly. Some ventilators have the clever option of allowing you to blow air down the circuit to dry it.

Key Point	Terminology	Practical Tip	Physiology	How to do it

Patients using NIV at home tend not to get infections from dirty circuits. Their equipment needs to look clean, but it doesn't need to be sterile.

Filters

We need to put a bacterial filter at the ventilator end of the circuit to protect the ventilator (Figure 11.8). Since air is always blowing one way up the tubing, bacteria can't get much more than about 10 cm upstream from the exhalation port. However, if some water condenses in the circuit or if the patient coughs some sputum into the tubing, it is possible for these liquids to run back into the ventilator by gravity if the patient end of the circuit is higher. The inside of a ventilator is very difficult to sterilise, so as a precaution put in a filter to protect it. Make sure you use a simple (thin) bacterial filter, not a heat and moisture exchanger (HME) which would increase the resistance to flow, particularly when wet. The outside of the ventilator should be wiped down regularly to keep it clean.

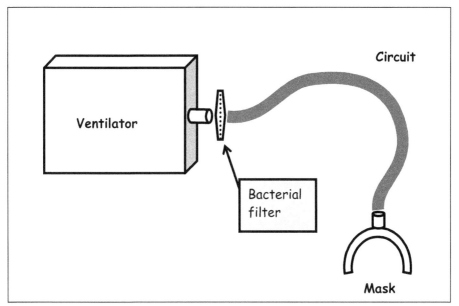

Figure 11.8 A bacterial filter is placed on the ventilator outlet, to prevent the inside becoming contaminated.

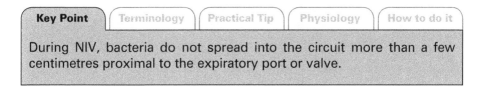

Key Point | Terminology | Practical Tip | Physiology | How to do it

During NIV, bacteria do not spread into the circuit more than a few centimetres proximal to the expiratory port or valve.

Safety Valves

You may come across safety valves incorporated into the circuit. The purpose of these is to allow the patient to breathe if the ventilator stops working. These have holes which are closed off by small flaps when the circuit is pressurised, which fall back to open the holes if the ventilator doesn't generate any pressure.

They are not needed if the patient is using a nasal mask, or if they would be able to remove the mask themselves if there was a problem.

Key Point	Terminology	**Practical Tip**	Physiology	How to do it

Bi-level circuits sometimes have swivel connectors, safety valves (to allow the patient to breathe if the ventilator fails), pressure monitoring ports, oxygen connectors etc. It is easy to mistake these for an exhalation port.

Summary

- The circuit for bi-level NIV is a large tube, with a small hole near the patient end, out of which exhaled air escapes
- A bacterial filter at the other end stops the ventilator from becoming contaminated
- Circuits for some NIV ventilators have an exhalation valve, which is closed during inspiration by pressure supplied through a separate small bore tube

12
Inspiratory Pressure

Learning points

By the end of this chapter you should be able to:

- Decide when to increase IPAP
- Define span
- Describe rise time and when to reduce it
- Explain how compliance affects NIV

We have noted already that when you blow air into a patient's lungs with a ventilator, the harder you blow (i.e. the more IPAP) the more air you will get in (Figure 12.1). Earlier, when you started a patient on bi-level pressure-support we used 12 to 15 cmH_2O for the IPAP, but for pressure-control we started with 20 cmH_2O.

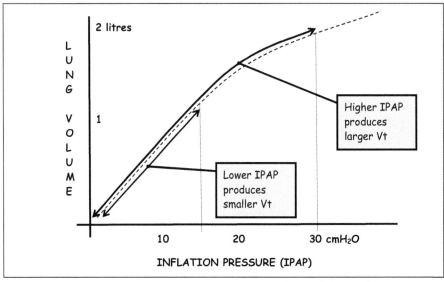

Figure 12.1 Pressure-volume curve showing that a higher IPAP produces a larger tidal volume.

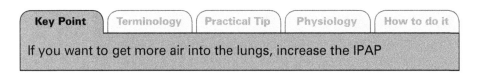

| Key Point | Terminology | Practical Tip | Physiology | How to do it |

If you want to get more air into the lungs, increase the IPAP

Here are a few points about IPAP:
- **Higher pressures produce a higher Vt. If your patient gets used to NIV but their blood gases don't improve, try increasing the pressure**
- **Increasing IPAP may also increase leaks (and so decrease tolerance of NIV)**
- **If your patient is using supplementary oxygen, on increasing IPAP you will blow more oxygen out of the expiratory port — to keep the same FiO$_2$, you may need to increase the oxygen flow rate**
- **You won't be able to get inspiratory pressures much above 30 cmH$_2$O because the mask blows off the face**
- **An IPAP of less than 10 cmH$_2$O provides very little assistance to ventilation**
- **If you increase IPAP, you may need to increase inspiratory time, to allow time for more air to flow into the lungs.**

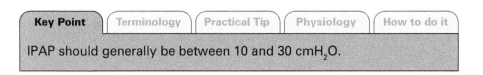

| Key Point | Terminology | Practical Tip | Physiology | How to do it |

IPAP should generally be between 10 and 30 cmH$_2$O.

IPAP and span

Span is a term you may come across which is used for the difference between IPAP and EPAP. Vt depends on this difference.

Let's look at span for single level and bi-level NIV, with both set at an IPAP of 15 cmH$_2$O. When there is no expiratory pressure, the pressure swings between 0 and 15 cmH$_2$O. With bi-level NIV we often use an EPAP of 5 cmH$_2$O; the difference between this and an IPAP of 15 cmH$_2$O is 10 cmH$_2$O (Figure 12.2). Increase the EPAP to 10 cmH$_2$O and the difference between this and the IPAP — "span" — is only 5 cmH$_2$O. You may hear the terms "low span" and "high span" used in ICU.

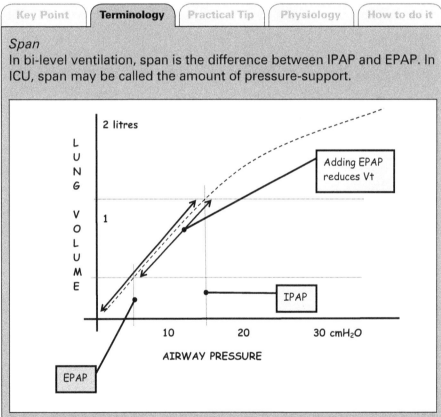

Key Point | **Terminology** | **Practical Tip** | **Physiology** | **How to do it**

Span
In bi-level ventilation, span is the difference between IPAP and EPAP. In ICU, span may be called the amount of pressure-support.

Figure 12.2 Pressure-volume curve of the lungs, showing the Vt obtained with IPPV and an IPAP of 15 cmH$_2$O; or with bi-level pressure-control 15/5 (i.e. the same IPAP but with an EPAP of 5 cmH$_2$O).

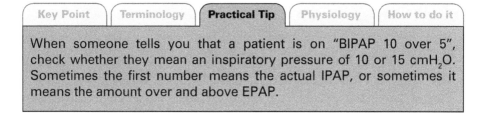

| Key Point | Terminology | **Practical Tip** | Physiology | How to do it |

When someone tells you that a patient is on "BIPAP 10 over 5", check whether they mean an inspiratory pressure of 10 or 15 cmH$_2$O. Sometimes the first number means the actual IPAP, or sometimes it means the amount over and above EPAP.

Rise time

Some ventilators have the facility to adjust "rise time" (or "ramp"). Usually you won't have to worry about this, but now would be a good time just to explain what it means. When the ventilator triggers into inspiration, it takes a little while for it to reach the target IPAP, particularly if you are using higher pressures. So if the respiratory rate is very fast the patient won't get the IPAP you intended. One way of correcting this problem is to shorten the rise time, if this facility is available on your ventilator (Figure 12.3).

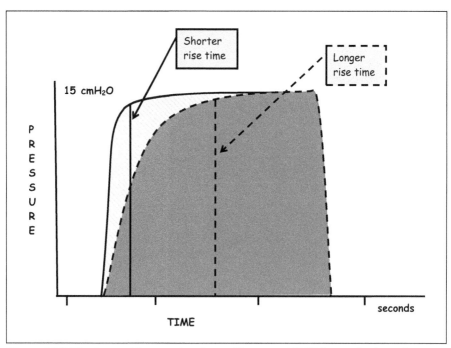

Figure 12.3 Shorter and longer rise times. The target IPAP is reached much sooner with a shorter rise time.

In practice, you don't usually need to worry about rise time, except in patients with very high respiratory drive who are breathing very fast. It is worth just looking at the pressure indicator on the ventilator (on the graphical display or other indicator) to check that the target pressure is being reached by the end of inspiration. Shortening the rise time may help with this.

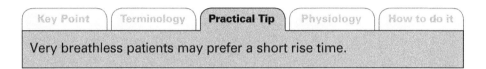

| Key Point | Terminology | **Practical Tip** | Physiology | How to do it |

Very breathless patients may prefer a short rise time.

| Key Point | Terminology | Practical Tip | **Physiology** | How to do it |

Work of breathing
To get air into the lungs, the inspiratory muscles use energy. This energy is needed to overcome two different factors — the "elastic" tendency of the lungs to collapse like a balloon, and the "resistance" to flow of air down the airways (Figure 12.4).

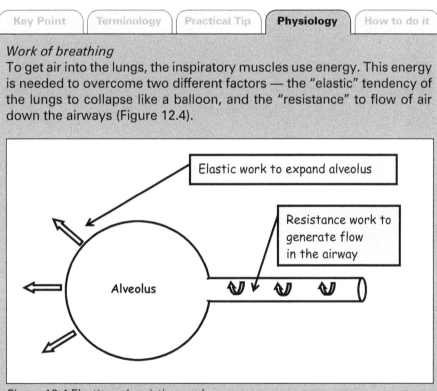

Elastic work to expand alveolus

Resistance work to generate flow in the airway

Alveolus

Figure 12.4 Elastic and resistive work.

"Elastic" work is much greater if the lungs or chest wall are less compliant (i.e. stiffer). Taking small breaths takes less work, so these patients will choose a fast respiratory rate with a small Vt (Figure 12.5).

cont ...

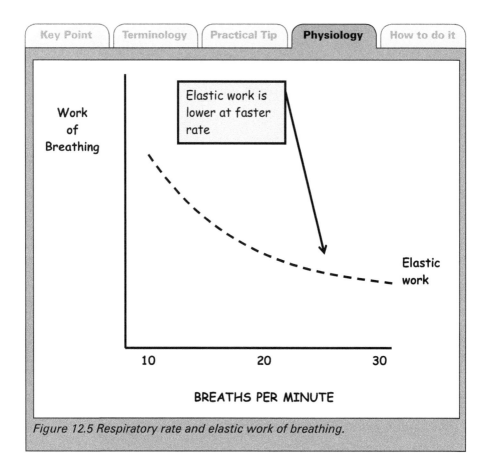

| Key Point | Terminology | Practical Tip | **Physiology** | How to do it |

Figure 12.5 Respiratory rate and elastic work of breathing.

Summary

- **More IPAP means more ventilation**
- **In bi-level NIV, increasing EPAP will reduce ventilation by reducing span**
- **Check that the patient is actually getting the pressure you have set**
- **Occasionally you may need to shorten the rise time in a very breathless patient**

13
Chronic Obstructive Pulmonary Disease

Learning points

By the end of this chapter you should be able to:

- **Decide when to start a patient with COPD on NIV**
- **Connect oxygen or a nebuliser to NIV**
- **Explain why supplementary oxygen may be harmful in COPD**
- **Discuss which COPD patients might benefit from long-term NIV**

Patients who need NIV acutely can be split into two main groups:

1. Those with common diseases such as COPD who present with acute hypercapnic respiratory failure and need NIV for a few hours or days during the acute illness. Their pH level will be low.
2. Those with fairly normal lungs who slip into hypercapnic respiratory failure because their breathing muscles give up or their central respiratory drive is poor (ventilatory pump failure). Their pH level may be normal. Many of these patients will need long-term NIV at home. Sometimes you get warning signs that trouble is brewing and can start NIV electively, but quite often there is a crisis and NIV is started acutely.

In this chapter we'll look at the commonest situation in which NIV is needed — an acute exacerbation of COPD.

Which COPD patients?

NIV is not indicated in an acute exacerbation of COPD if the patient does not have a respiratory acidosis. Perhaps the commonest mistake in NIV is to use it in a patient with COPD whose pH level is greater than 7.35. If the patient does become acidotic, NIV can be used much earlier than intubation in the course of the exacerbation to break the downward spiral into increasingly severe acidosis.

| Key Point | Terminology | Practical Tip | Physiology | How to do it |

In acute exacerbations of COPD, only use NIV in patients with a respiratory acidosis (pH <7.35).

| Key Point | Terminology | Practical Tip | **Physiology** | How to do it |

Acute-on-chronic type 2 respiratory failure
In Figure 6.7 we noted that retention of bicarbonate creates a new line on our $PaCO_2$-pH graph if there is chronic type 2 respiratory failure. If the $PaCO_2$ climbs further in an exacerbation, our patient travels up the new line (Figure 13.1). An acute-on-chronic respiratory acidosis is a high $PaCO_2$, low pH and high HCO_3^-.

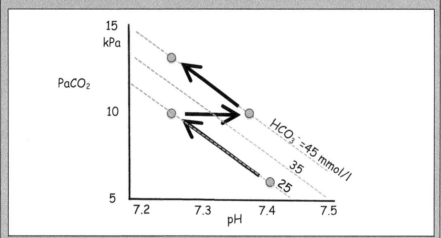

Figure 13.1 In an acute respiratory acidosis, as $PaCO_2$ rises our patient travels along the 25 mmol/l bicarbonate line and the pH falls. With renal retention of bicarbonate, the pH returns to normal, despite a high $PaCO_2$. We are now on the 45 mmol/l line, and will travel up this line if the $PaCO_2$ rises further: an acute-on-chronic respiratory acidosis.

Before you have to decide whether or not to use NIV, you will usually have time to administer drug therapy — such as nebulised bronchodilators — and set up properly controlled oxygen therapy. After an hour or so, if things are not improving then it is time for NIV. By this time you should have had a chance to move the patient to HDU, or a similar area where NIV is used regularly.

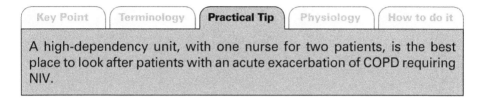

| Key Point | Terminology | **Practical Tip** | Physiology | How to do it |

A high-dependency unit, with one nurse for two patients, is the best place to look after patients with an acute exacerbation of COPD requiring NIV.

Some patients are so sick that you should intubate them and ventilate them invasively: these patients are usually more acidotic. Severe acidosis in itself does not preclude a trial of NIV if it is safe to do so; you may have to start NIV sooner — in the Emergency Department or Acute Medicine Unit — but the patient needs to be transferred to ICU as soon as possible.

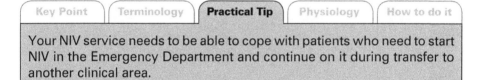

| Key Point | Terminology | **Practical Tip** | Physiology | How to do it |

Your NIV service needs to be able to cope with patients who need to start NIV in the Emergency Department and continue on it during transfer to another clinical area.

Choosing the right patients

There are a number of things which might make you choose intubation rather than NIV:

- If there is evidence of pneumonia on the chest X-ray, the chances of NIV succeeding are greatly reduced
- The more abnormal the physiology, the less likely NIV is to work. There are a number of scoring systems which you may be familiar with. The single most important factor for decisions about NIV is systolic hypotension
- Be wary of using NIV in patients with altered conscious level

- Thin COPD patients don't tend to do terribly well on NIV, but it is still worth a trial. The reason for this is not clear, but my interpretation is that these thin patients are "pink puffers" with high respiratory drives who are not normally hypercapnic; the fact that they have slipped into type 2 respiratory failure indicates that they have run out of functioning lung surface area and are nearing the end of their life
- If the patient is breathing very fast — above 30/min — they may struggle with NIV. It's worth a try, since some patients will settle to a lower rate quite quickly. If they don't, they might be better with invasive ventilation

Ventilator settings

As we've already mentioned, bi-level pressure-support is the best mode for COPD. Start with an IPAP of 12 cmH_2O and an EPAP of 5 cmH_2O. Push up the IPAP slowly towards 20 cmH_2O during the course of the next few hours depending on the response. To correct hypercapnia you may even need to go up to 30 cmH_2O, but in COPD you should start fairly low and build the IPAP up. (For some reason, breathless COPD patients often really struggle to tolerate NIV if you start with a decent IPAP, hence the approach of starting with a modest pressure and building it up. In contrast, neuromuscular, obesity-hypoventilation and scoliosis patients get the hang of NIV more quickly if you start with a higher IPAP, perhaps because it is then easier for them to relax and let the ventilator do all the work — starting with a low IPAP and building up is the wrong thing to do for them. This difference in approach is, of course, not applicable to every patient — some COPD patients will tolerate a high IPAP straight away, and some non-COPD patients struggle even with a low IPAP.)

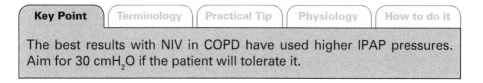

| Key Point | Terminology | **Practical Tip** | Physiology | How to do it |

NIV ventilators designed for home use are OK for acute exacerbations of COPD, but a more sophisticated "HDU" ventilator with an integral oxygen blender will work much better.

We'll see in the chapter on triggering (Chapter 26) why it may be necessary to increase the EPAP slightly, but not above 10 cmH$_2$O. Set the back-up rate to about 12 breaths per minute, with an inspiratory:expiratory ratio of 1:3 for these breaths, to leave the patient plenty of time to breathe out — more of this in the chapter on I:E ratios (Chapter 32).

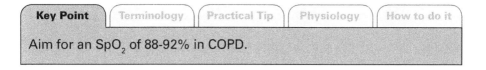

| **Key Point** | Terminology | Practical Tip | Physiology | How to do it |

The best results with NIV in COPD have used higher IPAP pressures. Aim for 30 cmH$_2$O if the patient will tolerate it.

Oxygen

If the oxygen saturation is below 88% once the patient is established on NIV, add supplemental oxygen, starting at 1 l/min and increasing until the saturation runs between 88 and 92%. If you give too much oxygen they will stop breathing, leaving NIV to provide all the ventilation, which may not be enough.

| **Key Point** | Terminology | Practical Tip | Physiology | How to do it |

Aim for an SpO$_2$ of 88-92% in COPD.

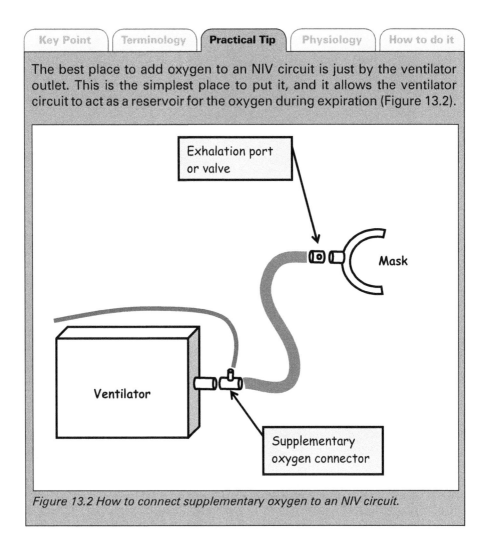

The best place to add oxygen to an NIV circuit is just by the ventilator outlet. This is the simplest place to put it, and it allows the ventilator circuit to act as a reservoir for the oxygen during expiration (Figure 13.2).

Exhalation port or valve

Mask

Ventilator

Supplementary oxygen connector

Figure 13.2 How to connect supplementary oxygen to an NIV circuit.

Duration of NIV

If after one hour of NIV the acidosis is not improving, you should consider abandoning NIV and intubating the patient. You may have time to adjust the ventilator settings (mainly by increasing the IPAP) and re-assess after another hour or so, but if there has been no improvement after 4 hours then NIV is probably not doing any good and should be stopped. Aim for NIV most of the time for the first 24 hours, accepting that in practice the patient will only spend about 15 hours on the ventilator by the time they have had breaks for nebulisers, meals etc. The next day you can plan longer breaks, but they will probably still use NIV overnight. By the day after that, the patient will normally be better and probably refusing to use NIV anyway.

Key Point	Terminology	Practical Tip	Physiology	How to do it

It will usually be apparent from checking arterial blood gases after about an hour of NIV whether or not it is going to work in acute respiratory failure.

Long term

There are trials in progress to see whether NIV using high inflation pressures, titrated to correct nocturnal hypoventilation, will benefit a wider group of patients with COPD in the longer term. For the moment, here are some reasons why you might want to use NIV at home in COPD:

• **Recurrent episodes of respiratory acidosis**
  Longer-term NIV is needed in only a small proportion of patients with COPD. If the patient has had more than three exacerbations requiring NIV within the last six months (and has tolerated NIV well), then you should consider leaving them on it at night at home indefinitely. These patients are usually obese with poor respiratory drive, and probably overlap with the obesity-hypoventilation syndrome. Ask the patient — success is more likely if they are keen to use NIV and feel it does them some good.

• **Nocturnal hypoventilation with sleep disturbance**
  We all have a slightly higher $PaCO_2$ at night than during the day, reflecting lower alveolar ventilation during sleep. Patients with daytime hypercapnia will always be worse during sleep. If this causes them to wake up frequently during the night, they can experience excessive sleepiness during the daytime. A trial of NIV may be warranted to see if it improves their sleepiness. After a month or so, let the patient decide if they want to continue with it.

• **Long-term oxygen**
  Sometimes NIV is the only way you can establish a patient with COPD on long-term oxygen therapy without inducing dangerous hypercapnia. There are no hard-and-fast rules about this, but use the lowest FiO_2 which gets the PaO_2 above 8 kPa — if this causes the $PaCO_2$ to rise above 10 kPa then it is probably safer to use NIV (in combination with oxygen.)

Key Point | Terminology | Practical Tip | **Physiology** | How to do it

Resistive work of breathing

When you apply IPAP, the patient's lung may not simply travel up and down the pressure-volume curve we are becoming familiar with. If there is significant resistance to flow, the pressure increases but there isn't much flow. Once the air starts to flow, volume increases. When we reach the end of inspiration, there is no longer any flow. No flow means no pressure drop from resistance. We're back where we should be on the curve (Figure 13.3). This bowed curve is the "dynamic" compliance, as opposed to the "static" compliance dictated only by elastic forces.

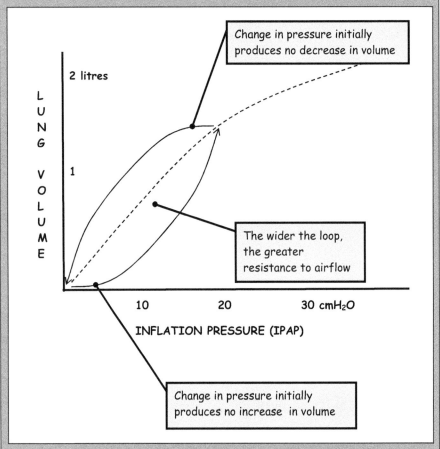

Figure 13.3 Dynamic compliance. The work done by the ventilator (or inspiratory muscles) to inflate the lungs can be sub-divided into elastic and resistive work.

cont ...

| Key Point | Terminology | Practical Tip | **Physiology** | How to do it |

Resistive work is greater when high flow rates are generated. It is lowest with a long slow breath (Figure 13.4).

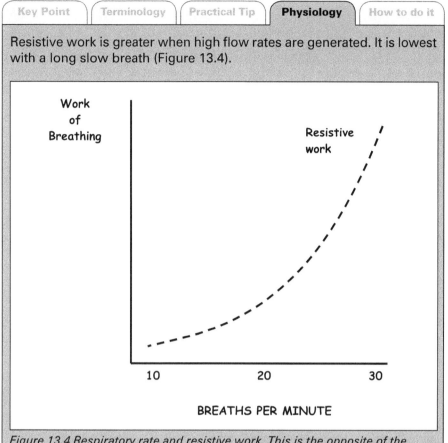

Figure 13.4 Respiratory rate and resistive work. This is the opposite of the curve we saw for patients with high elastic work (Figure 12.5).

Summary

- In acute exacerbations of COPD, NIV helps patients with an acute respiratory acidosis (pH <7.35)
- If you need to add oxygen or a nebuliser, position it near the ventilator outlet
- Very few patients with COPD need NIV long-term

14
Weaning from NIV

Learning points

By the end of this chapter you should be able to:

- Decide when to stop NIV in a patient who is getting better from acute respiratory failure
- Describe how you would wean from daytime NIV
- Give an example of when you might discontinue NIV in a patient who has been on it long-term at home

Many patients with an acute exacerbation of COPD will decide for themselves when they no longer need NIV and will refuse to use it. This is usually fine, but monitor them overnight for the first night just to be sure that they are going to be OK.

Other patients will take a bit longer, and may become psychologically dependent on NIV. The best way to wean them is to gradually increase the length of periods of spontaneous breathing: this works better than turning down the pressure on the ventilator. You will probably want to keep them on NIV overnight for a few nights, but aim to have them breathing spontaneously all day as soon as they can. Then just stop nocturnal NIV, monitoring overnight for the first night and re-assess the following morning.

Key Point

Wean patients from NIV by lengthening their periods of spontaneous ventilation, not by reducing the NIV pressures.

Weaning to long-term nocturnal NIV

For patients with conditions that are likely to need long-term NIV, your aim may be to wean to spontaneous ventilation during the day, but continue with nocturnal NIV indefinitely. Examples of such patients would be patients with obesity, scoliosis or neuromuscular problems who presented with acute respiratory failure. The principles of establishing spontaneous ventilation during the daytime are the same.

Before you start to wean, you need to be sure that you are providing adequate ventilation with NIV. If the $PaCO_2$ is still high on NIV, you are not achieving your aim. Things you could do, usually in this in order, are:

- **Increase the IPAP**
- **Change to pressure-control**
- **Lengthen inspiratory time**
- **Increase the rate**

Once the $PaCO_2$ is normal, then you can think about trials of spontaneous ventilation.

It also helps if you can get the bicarbonate down to normal. Normalising $PaCO_2$ should do this, but a daily dose of acetazolamide will speed things up.

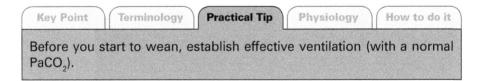

Key Point | Terminology | **Practical Tip** | Physiology | How to do it

Before you start to wean, establish effective ventilation (with a normal $PaCO_2$).

| Key Point | Terminology | Practical Tip | Physiology | **How to do it** |

Wean from NIV to spontaneous ventilation
- Explain to the patient what you are planning to do and why
- When you are sure that they understand and agree with your plan, stop NIV
- Stay by the patient
- Give them supplementary oxygen if they are likely to desaturate — this is quite safe just for a few minutes.
- Watch them breathe. Make sure they can achieve some chest expansion, particularly in patients with neuromuscular conditions — if not, re-start NIV and think again
- The respiratory rate may be high initially, but will fall within a few minutes. Don't put the patient back on the ventilator just because they look "tired" or anxious. Persevere, stay with them and they may settle down with reassurance.
- The length of the first spontaneous breathing trial will vary. Some will only manage five minutes, but it is still an important step — make each subsequent trial slightly longer. Others will stay off for hours quite happily

There should be a daily plan, in which the amount of ventilatory support is reviewed and clear goals set. Every day you should ask yourself why your patient is still on a ventilator. Then decide what the minimum support from NIV that they need is and make a plan accordingly. Aim low. You can always step back up if the patient starts to struggle — it is a common mistake to have patients on more support than they need.

| Key Point | Terminology | **Practical Tip** | Physiology | How to do it |

In patients with chronic lung disease, remember that their blood gases may be terrible even when they are stable and "well". If you aim for a normal PaO_2 it will take you ages to get them off ventilation.

Weaning from nocturnal NIV in hospital

Once your patient is happy to breathe all day by themselves, decide if there is any reason to think that long-term nocturnal NIV will be the best option for them. It often will be, for example with scoliosis, obesity or neuromuscular problems. Even if the underlying neurological disease seems to have responded to treatment, for example in myasthenia gravis, it is usually safer to settle for nocturnal NIV for a few months at home.

If everything is going well and you don't think nocturnal NIV is needed any more, just stop it. Keep the ventilator by the bedside at least for the first night, so that the patient knows it is there in case they need to go back onto it. Obviously you'll want to monitor closely and re-assess the situation carefully the next morning.

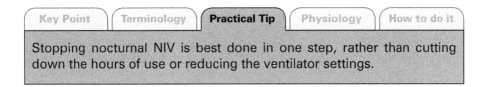

| Key Point | Terminology | **Practical Tip** | Physiology | How to do it |

Stopping nocturnal NIV is best done in one step, rather than cutting down the hours of use or reducing the ventilator settings.

Weaning from nocturnal NIV at home

Patients who have a ventilator at home but don't need it usually take things into their own hands and use it only intermittently, if at all. Just look at the hours of use.

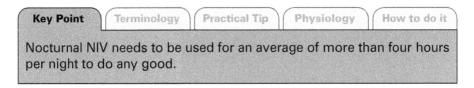

| **Key Point** | Terminology | Practical Tip | Physiology | How to do it |

Nocturnal NIV needs to be used for an average of more than four hours per night to do any good.

The patient may want to try stopping NIV if the original problem has resolved, for example polymyositis that has improved with drug therapy or if an obese patient has lost a significant amount of weight. As with nocturnal NIV in hospital, the best thing to do is just stop it rather than cutting down the hours of use or reducing the pressures. If this is the wrong decision, it will take about three weeks for the patient to starting running into problems. This can be a worrying time for the patient, so I see them every week in the out-patient clinic. It is seldom necessary or productive to admit the patient to hospital for observation whilst you withdraw NIV.

| Key Point | Terminology | **Practical Tip** | Physiology | How to do it |

After stopping nocturnal NIV, see the patient in clinic every week for three weeks and check their arterial blood gas.

| Key Point | Terminology | Practical Tip | **Physiology** | How to do it |

Respiratory muscle fatigue
Muscles get fatigued if they are asked to do too much work with insufficient time for recovery between each contraction. Imagine if you were asked to lift a really heavy weight once an hour; you might be able to manage it, but what would happen if you had to lift it every thirty seconds?

For the respiratory muscles, we can calculate the tension time index. The first part of the equation is inspiratory time as a fraction of total breath time — if a high proportion of the total breath time is taken up by inspiration, there isn't much time for the muscles to recover before the next breath in. The second part of the equation is the load/capacity balance we have discussed before — the force generated during each breath in, as a proportion of the maximum strength of the inspiratory muscles:

$$\text{tension-time index} = \frac{\text{inspiratory time}}{\text{total breath time}} \times \frac{\text{tidal inspiratory pressure}}{\text{maximum inspiratory pressure}}$$

The tidal inspiratory pressure is quite difficult to measure, unless you have a pressure probe in the oesophagus, but we could use the ratio of tidal volume to vital capacity:

$$\frac{\text{inspiratory time}}{\text{total breath time}} \times \frac{\text{tidal volume}}{\text{vital capacity}}$$

It doesn't really matter what the critical value of the tension-time Index is, but it is important to understand the concept that the timing of breathing and the proportion of maximum available force used are both key determinants of muscle fatigue.

Summary

- The best way to wean from NIV is to use progressively longer spontaneous breathing trials, rather than reducing pressures
- Weaning from nocturnal NIV is best done as a single step

15
Respiratory Rate

Learning points

By the end of this chapter you should be able to:

• Describe how back-up rate works for a patient on pressure-support
• Describe how respiratory rate affects the work of breathing
• Set respiratory rate for pressure-control

Bi-level pressure-support

Most of the time, a patient on pressure-support will dictate their own respiratory rate. If they were to stop breathing (for example a patient with chronic respiratory failure who is given too much oxygen) then we want the ventilator to kick in with a back-up rate. Common settings are about 10-15 breaths per minute. Fifteen breaths per minute mean one breath every four seconds. In Figure 15.1, the patient stops breathing after the third breath; when four seconds have elapsed, the back-up rate of the ventilator kicks in (set to 15 breaths per minute in this example). Sometimes these breaths initiated by the ventilator are called mandatory or control breaths.

111

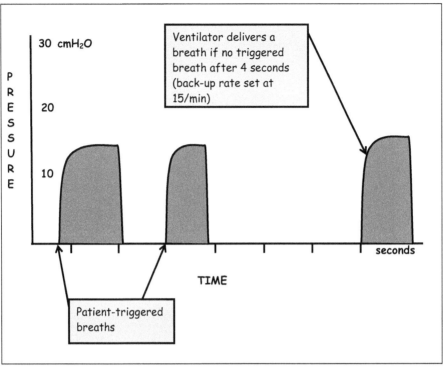

Figure 15.1 In bi-level pressure-support, respiratory rate refers to the back-up rate at which the ventilator will deliver a breath if the patient stops breathing.

If the patient does not improve on your initial settings, one possible way of improving ventilation is to increase the back-up rate until the ventilator is going faster than the patient's spontaneous rate. In practice, playing around with the back-up settings on a pressure-support ventilator seldom seems to do much for gas exchange, perhaps because that is not what the ventilator was primarily designed to do. If you really want to dictate what sort of breath is delivered, use pressure-control.

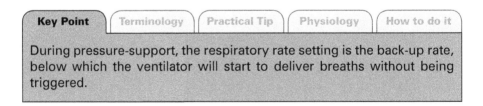

Key Point | Terminology | Practical Tip | **Physiology** | How to do it

Respiratory rate

Faster rates with smaller volumes mean less "elastic" work of breathing and less energy expended in stretching the lungs and ribcage (like stretching an elastic band) with each breath.

There are two problems with fast respiratory rates:

- A greater proportion of the small volume breaths is wasted on dead-space
- More ventilation goes to "fast" alveoli with short time constants. We'll look at this point later

Slower rates mean less "resistance" work pushing air in and out of the airways, because there is more time for air to get into the lungs and so flow rates are lower.

The total work of breathing is the sum of elastic and resistance work. Patients automatically choose the best rate for their particular combination of compliance and resistance, to minimise the amount of energy they use in breathing (Figure 15.2).

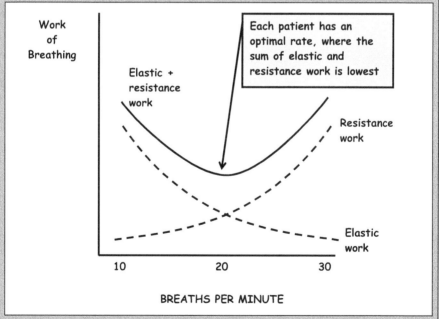

Figure 15.2 Total work of breathing at different respiratory rates.

Pressure-control

With pressure-control, the ventilator determines the timing of each breath as well as the target pressure. Set the rate at, or just below, the patient's own rate. This will often be quite fast, but if you try and start with a slower rate, the patient will probably struggle to co-ordinate with the ventilator. The rate can be slowed down as the patient's clinical condition improves.

Summary

- **With pressure-support you don't need to worry too much about respiratory rate, but set a reasonable back-up rate**
- **When starting pressure-control, set the respiratory rate at the patient's own spontaneous rate. Slow the rate down gradually**

16
Sequelae of Tuberculosis

Learning points

By the end of this chapter you should be able to:

- **Give examples of pre-chemotherapy treatments for TB which increase the risk of respiratory failure**
- **Describe what to look for in a patient with old TB who might have slipped into hypercapnic respiratory failure**

Prior to the discovery of anti-tuberculous chemotherapy, treatment for tuberculosis sometimes involved a phrenic nerve crush, artificial pneumothorax or thoracoplasty. These procedures, combined with the inevitable lung damage from the infection itself, left patients with a high work of breathing and/or impaired respiratory muscle pump. Many of these patients slip into hypercapnic respiratory failure as a late complication decades later.

Risk of ventilatory failure

Any patient who had a thoracoplasty is at high risk of slipping into hypercapnic respiratory failure as they get older. Effective anti-tuberculous drugs became available in the 1950s, with the number of operations declining rapidly thereafter. There are only a very small numbers of these patients around still, so seeing them every year in clinic is not a large burden.

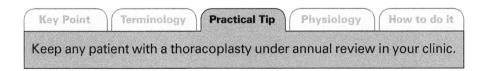

| Key Point | Terminology | **Practical Tip** | Physiology | How to do it |

Keep any patient with a thoracoplasty under annual review in your clinic.

It's probably worth keeping an eye on those that had a pneumonectomy also, since it is highly likely that their remaining lung will have been damaged by the original infection. If they just had a phrenic nerve crush or lobectomy then check the VC and if it is above 1.5 litres then you could tell them what to watch out for and give them an open appointment.

Non-invasive ventilation

As with scoliosis, nocturnal NIV should be commenced if a patient with a thoracoplasty is hypercapnic, irrespective of the pH level. NIV is reasonably effective at improving their clinical condition and blood gases, but long-term survival rates are poor. NIV should be set up as for scoliosis (IPPV, decent IPAP, rate similar to the patient's spontaneous rate), except that the presence of airflow obstruction from endobronchial tuberculous scarring will usually require a slightly longer expiratory time when you set the I:E ratio. The inevitable damage to the lungs from extensive tuberculosis means that supplementary oxygen is often necessary.

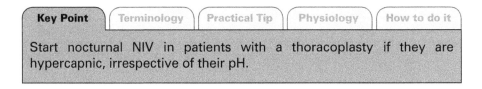

| **Key Point** | Terminology | Practical Tip | Physiology | How to do it |

Start nocturnal NIV in patients with a thoracoplasty if they are hypercapnic, irrespective of their pH.

Summary

- There are still some patients around who are at risk of developing ventilatory failure as a consequence of surgical procedures for TB
- Keep these patients under annual review in your out-patient clinic
- Start NIV as soon the $PaCO_2$ rises above 6 kPa

17
Non-Invasive or Invasive?

Learning points

By the end of this chapter you should be able to:

- Decide which patients should be intubated straight away rather than managed with NIV
- Discuss how you would decide whether or not to proceed to intubation if your patient does not improve on NIV

We try to avoid intubating patients if we possibly can for the following reasons:

- The need for sedation means that getting back to spontaneous breathing may be a problem
- The patient cannot eat, so artificial feeding will be needed
- Hospital-acquired pneumonia is a worry
- Other complications may develop in ICU
- ICU beds are scarce

Nevertheless, there are some patients for whom intubation is a better option than NIV right from the start. There are others who may not do well on NIV and we need to resort to intubation in order to ventilate them properly. On the other hand, it is inappropriate to intubate if there is no possibility of the patient surviving. How do we identify those who are not going to do well?

Immediate intubation rather than NIV

Intubation is usually better than NIV for patients with any of the following:

- **Impaired conscious level – score <7 on the Glasgow Coma Scale (GCS)**
- **Multi-organ failure**
- **Severe hypoxia**
- **Respiratory arrest**
- **Total ventilator dependence**
- **Fixed upper airway obstruction**
- **Facial burns/trauma**
- **Head trauma/cerebrospinal fluid (CSF) leaks**
- **Sinus/middle ear infection**
- **Copious sputum production**

Most of the reasons are self-explanatory, but let's look at a few critical points in more detail.

Airway protection

If a patient on NIV vomits, there is a risk that they may inhale the vomit into their lungs. This is a big worry in an unconscious patient. If you vomit, you contract your laryngeal muscles to close your vocal cords tight shut. You don't take a breath in until you have cleared all the vomit from your throat. If anything does go down the wrong way into your lungs, you cough and splutter until it comes out again. An unconscious patient on NIV may vomit or regurgitate gastric contents into their pharynx. When the ventilator applies a positive pressure, gastric contents are pushed down into the lungs. The result is aspiration pneumonia. Some conscious patients with poor laryngeal muscle function, for example after a stroke or in motor neurone disease, may also be unable to protect their airway from aspiration during NIV.

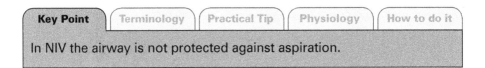

Key Point	Terminology	Practical Tip	Physiology	How to do it

In NIV the airway is not protected against aspiration.

Safe ventilation

On ICU, a ventilated patient has their endotracheal or tracheostomy tube secured in place with ties (or sometimes stitches in the case of a tracheostomy tube). The patient is usually pretty immobile, and so the chances of the ventilator becoming disconnected are low. In contrast, a patient on NIV is conscious and able to move their head; their ventilator is attached by some straps fastened with Velcro, and the mask can become displaced. If the patient is unable to breathe spontaneously at all, then disconnection could be disastrous, so close supervision of these patients is required (on HDU or ICU).

Effective ventilation

With invasive ventilation, inflation pressures up to 60 cmH$_2$O are sometimes used to ventilate patients with very stiff lungs or tight airways. With NIV, pressures much above 30 cmH$_2$O cause the mask to blow off the face of the patient, resulting in intolerable leaks. This is good in that barotrauma (damage caused by high inflation pressures) to the lung is not going to be a problem, but it does mean that some patients will need to be intubated in order to get higher inflation pressures.

With many smaller NIV ventilators without oxygen blenders, it is impossible to get the inspired oxygen concentration above 30%. If the patient has such a severe problem with gas exchange that they need more oxygen than this, they will need to be intubated.

During NIV, the patient is awake and breathing with their own rhythm, or something pretty close. When they are sedated and intubated you have much more scope to play around with the timing of respiration in order to try and improve gas exchange.

Secretions

Every time a patient wants to cough out secretions from their lungs, they need to take off their mask. This is fine if it only happens every few minutes, but if they have a very productive cough — for example in bronchiectasis — then they will spend all the time taking the mask on and off and derive no benefit from the ventilator. Intubation will probably be a better option if the patient is coughing up sputum most of the time.

Intubate the patient on the basis of their clinical condition, taking into account their arterial blood gas values — not on the blood gas values alone.

NIV for patients who are not for intubation

If you decide in advance that intubation is not an option, there is nothing to stop you trying NIV in patients with any of the contraindications listed at the beginning of the chapter, for example an unconscious patient or someone with severe hypoxia. Most of these contra-indications are relative, rather than absolute. If you are aware of the potential complications you can take measures to minimise the risk. Do it in a safe place, like HDU, with a nurse-patient ratio of 1:2.

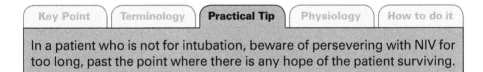

| Key Point | Terminology | **Practical Tip** | Physiology | How to do it |

In a patient who is not for intubation, beware of persevering with NIV for too long, past the point where there is any hope of the patient surviving.

| Key Point | Terminology | Practical Tip | Physiology | **How to do it** |

Ventilate an unconscious patient using NIV
• Keep the patient propped up in bed as high as you can
• Use a full-face mask
• Pass a nasogastric tube first
• Aspirate the nasogastric tube regularly to keep the stomach empty
• Start the patient on drugs to reduce gastric acidity, to minimise the chemical damage to the lungs if they do aspirate
• Aspirate pharyngeal secretions regularly

Intubation when NIV fails

A patient may deteriorate on NIV, and you have to decide whether to intubate or not. There are two crucial questions to ask:

• **Has it been possible to establish the patient on NIV?**
If the patient has failed to settle on NIV for some reason, for example because they cannot tolerate a mask, then they have not really had a trial of assisted ventilation. You need a different interface between the patient and the ventilator — an endotracheal tube — to see if ventilation is going to work. On the other hand, you may have settled the patient onto NIV fairly quickly, then increased the IPAP to 20 cmH$_2$O or so and added supplementary oxygen. If they fail to improve at this point then it is failure of assisted ventilation, rather than failure of NIV. Changing the interface to an endotracheal tube is going to make much less difference than in the patient who couldn't tolerate a mask — the rewards of intubation are likely to be lower.

• **Is the patient likely to survive intubation?**
This is a difficult decision and there isn't much decent quality data on which to base it. The bottom line is that patients often do much better than expected, and if in doubt they should be intubated. In patients with an acute exacerbation of COPD, there are a few factors which are commonly used to identify patients who don't do well:

  • No clear reversible reason for deterioration
  • Normal CXR. (No pneumonia or pneumothorax as a reversible cause for deterioration, implying that the patient has simply run out of functioning lung)
  • Presence of co-morbidities
  • Low body mass index
  • Poor exercise tolerance (housebound) prior to exacerbation

Key Point	Terminology	**Practical Tip**	Physiology	How to do it

Provided it is safe to do so, it is usually better to keep your NIV patients out of ICU. Staff in ICUs tend to feel more comfortable with invasive ventilation; the environment there can be pretty noisy; and day-night differentiation can be a problem for the patient's sleep clock.

Summary

- Intubation is a better option for unconscious patients who are unable to protect their own airway
- Careful monitoring in HDU or ICU is mandatory if NIV is used in patients who are unable to do at least some breathing for themselves
- Intubation is usually better than NIV for patients with severe hypoxia or multiple system failure
- Don't delay intubation by tinkering around for too long with NIV in a severely ill patient

18

Weaning from Endotracheal Intubation to NIV

Learning points

By the end of this chapter you should be able to:

- Describe when to extubate a patient onto NIV
- Explain how you would do this

Some patients don't breathe very well after an operation or general anaesthetic. Using NIV in these circumstances makes sense. There are still quite a few unanswered questions about which groups of patients it helps. We'll consider the different situations shortly, but what is clear is that if it is going to work you need to start it early.

Key Point	Terminology	Practical Tip	Physiology	How to do it

If you are going to use NIV post-operatively, start it as soon as possible after extubation — don't wait until the patient runs into trouble, as it is much less likely to be effective at that stage.

Respiratory pump problems and elective surgical procedures

Patients with respiratory pump problems who have had elective surgical procedures — for example a gastroplasty or insertion of a feeding enterostomy tube under general anaesthesia — are excellent candidates for post-operative NIV. Clearly, if the patient is already using NIV long-term, they will need it immediately post-op.

There are some patients who are not yet at the stage of needing long-term NIV who will struggle post-operatively because of the effects of sedation, pain, analgesia, having to be supine etc. This is fairly easy to predict, and you can spend some time pre-operatively getting the patient used to NIV. This will make things much easier post-op. An example would be a patient with severe scoliosis, but without evidence of diurnal respiratory failure or nocturnal hypoventilation, who is going to undergo corrective spinal surgery.

Use bi-level pressure-control with an oro-nasal mask. You may need a higher IPAP than you used in the pre-operative trial. Depending on the type of operation, you may need to add supplementary oxygen. Aim to use NIV continuously for the first 24 hours post-op, with increasing periods of spontaneous breathing during the next few days. Clearly this will depend upon the type of operation and the speed of the patient's recovery.

Key Point	Terminology	**Practical Tip**	Physiology	How to do it

Plan to use NIV immediately after extubation in an obese patient who is likely to need opiates for post-operative analgesia.

Early extubation

Most patients who have been ventilated invasively for any length of time, or in whom weaning delay is anticipated, will have had a tracheostomy. This is fine most of the time, but weaning someone from ventilation via a tracheostomy to NIV takes time and sometimes you never manage it, for example in a patient with respiratory muscle weakness and a poor cough.

If you get the chance to go straight from intubation to NIV then it is well worth considering, provided the trial of NIV can be done safely. I would opt for early extubation to NIV in patients with respiratory pump failure (muscle weakness, chest wall deformity, obesity-hypoventilation syndrome) who have been intubated and ventilated for an episode of severe acute respiratory failure, and whose blood gases rapidly return to normal. The day after intubation you sometimes see patients who are easy to ventilate, with low inflation pressures, and who are easy to oxygenate on a fairly low inspired oxygen concentration. This tells you that the lungs are in reasonable shape, and that the main problem on admission was the respiratory pump — muscle failure or a central drive problem.

The length of time patients with acute exacerbations of COPD need to be ventilated for is sometimes surprisingly short. After extubation, some patients steadily deteriorate and need to be re-intubated. In most instances the next step will be a tracheostomy. You could have one more attempt at extubation, starting NIV straight away, provided this can be done safely and there is no evidence of pneumonia or other organ failure.

Pre-requisites for transferring a patient to NIV are as follows:

- **Normal PaCO$_2$**
- **Normal arterial pH and bicarbonate**
- **Normal, or only moderately low, PaO$_2$**
- **Inspired oxygen concentration requirement less than 30%**
- **Inflation pressure less than 30 cmH$_2$O**
- **Minimal respiratory tract secretions**
- **Reasonable cough**
- **Apyrexial**
- **Stable cardiac rhythm**
- **No inotropic support**
- **Normal electrolytes**
- **Stable renal function**
- **No evidence of fluid overload**
- **Functional gastrointestinal tract**
- **Adequate nutrition**

If all the above conditions are satisfied, there are a few questions to ask yourself:

- **Will the patient wake up when you stop the sedation? We have already noted the dangers of NIV in impaired consciousness. An intubated patient you are thinking of extubating and starting on NIV is quite likely to be sedated. You will have to decide if they are likely to regain full consciousness after you stop the sedation. If not, then it will be safer to do a tracheostomy**
- **Is it likely that the patient will be able to breathe by themselves for at least a few minutes within the next 24 hours? Although the**

patient may need to be on NIV all the time initially, it is much safer if they are able to breathe spontaneously for at least a few minutes
- Are the conditions optimal? You might decide to delay if it would be safer to extubate first thing the next morning, or at another time when the staffing arrangements are more secure, or when there is less going on elsewhere in ICU

Key Point	Terminology	**Practical Tip**	Physiology	How to do it

Extubate at a time of day when there is plenty of support at hand, when the patient can be rapidly intubated again if NIV fails.

Key Point	Terminology	Practical Tip	Physiology	**How to do it**

Extubate and start NIV
- Choose a ventilator mode that best matches the settings of the invasive ventilator they are on. This is likely to be bi-level pressure-control
- Set the NIV ventilator to the same IPAP, EPAP, rate and I:E ratio as the invasive ventilator
- Connect the NIV ventilator to the endotracheal tube for a few minutes to check that you are able to ventilate the patient effectively
- Re-connect the patient to the invasive ventilator
- Check that all the equipment needed for re-intubation is by the bedside
- Select a suitable mask and straps
- Connect the NIV ventilator to the mask
- Turn sedation off, and wait for the patient to start waking up
- Aspirate the nasogastic tube and remove it
- Aspirate the pharynx
- Aspirate the endotracheal tube and remove it
- Aspirate the pharynx again
- Place the mask over the patient's face and start NIV
- Wait a few minutes
- Adjust the respiratory rate or IPAP on the ventilator if you need to
- Strap the mask in place

| Key Point | Terminology | **Practical Tip** | Physiology | How to do it |

Assume that everyone who has been ventilated for a few days or more is fluid overloaded. This will make it difficult to wean them, and they may develop pulmonary oedema (and therefore stiff lungs) when they are extubated.

Summary

- NIV can reduce extubation failure rates
- Start it early

19
Chest Wall Trauma

Learning points

By the end of this chapter you should be able to:

- Explain why patients with multiple rib fractures have such a high risk of developing respiratory failure
- Describe how to manage them

Multiple rib fractures are associated with a poor prognosis, particularly in the elderly. Aggressive pain management is essential if you are to avoid the patient developing pneumonia, and you may need invasive techniques such as intercostal blocks or an epidural.

Many patients will need intubation and invasive ventilation. There are a few, however, who may get by with NIV for a short period. As is often the case for patients who need NIV, an elevated $PaCO_2$ indentifies those who are running into trouble.

Key Point	Terminology	Practical Tip	Physiology	How to do it

Patients with multiple fractured ribs do badly. Manage them on HDU and start NIV if they become hypercapnic.

Key Point | Terminology | Practical Tip | **Physiology** | How to do it

Flail segments

If the ribs are broken in two places, the patient may have a flail segment. This is a bit of the chest wall that is floating freely. During inspiration, there must be a negative pressure inside the thorax. The flail segment will therefore be sucked inwards, whereas the rest of the ribcage is expanding outwards. You will sometimes see this paradoxical inward motion of the sternum if it is broken. It is also inevitable after a thoracoplasty, where the ribs have been removed (Figure 19.1).

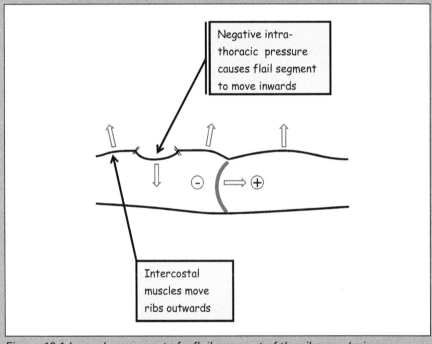

Figure 19.1 Inward movement of a flail segment of the ribcage during inspiration.

NIV

Although there isn't a great deal of evidence, there are good reasons for thinking that bi-level ventilation might help patients with multiple rib fractures who are slipping into ventilatory failure. If the pressure within the thorax is positive throughout the respiratory cycle, the flail segment shouldn't move as much (Figure 19.2). A bit of EPAP will help with atelectasis in the underlying lung, or in the bases if pain is preventing the patient from inhaling fully.

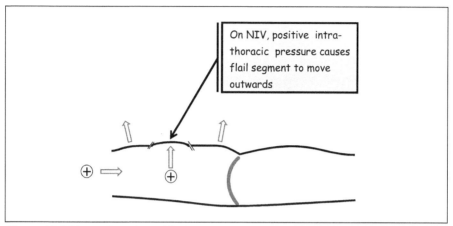

On NIV, positive intra-thoracic pressure causes flail segment to move outwards

Figure 19.2 Normal motion of flail segment on NIV.

Pressure-control should work best, if the patient is able to relax and allow the ventilator to do all the work. If they are unstable, with a fluctuating respiratory pattern, it may be easier to establish them on pressure-support. Start with the standard IPAP and EPAP of 12 and 5 cmH$_2$O respectively.

Start NIV early. This may help avoid intubation. The patient needs to be in a high dependency area. They need to be watched carefully. Move them to HDU or ICU.

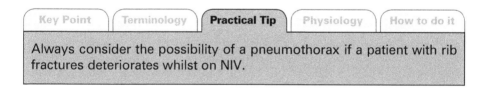

Key Point | Terminology | **Practical Tip** | Physiology | How to do it

Always consider the possibility of a pneumothorax if a patient with rib fractures deteriorates whilst on NIV.

Key Point Terminology Practical Tip **Physiology** How to do it

Intercostal muscle action

A bony ribcage is an essential part of the respiratory pump. The diaphragm needs a stable bony structure on which to pull, and the intercostals need hinged ribs to move up and down. Let's remind ourselves how they do this.

The external intercostals slope diagonally downwards. When they contract, they want to get shorter. (When your biceps contracts, your forearm moves up so that the muscle is shorter.) When your external intercostals contract, the ribs move upwards. In Figure 19.3 you can see how the distance between the two points of attachment of the muscle are shorter.

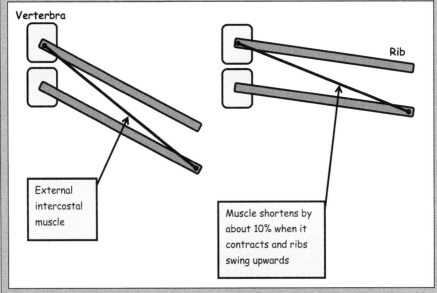

Figure 19.3 Movement of ribs upwards on inspiration, when external intercostal muscles contract.

Summary

- **NIV can work in carefully selected patients with multiple rib fractures**
- **Start it early**
- **Move the patient to HDU or ICU**

20
Monitoring

Learning points

By the end of this chapter you should be able to:

* Set up monitoring for a patient with acute respiratory failure on NIV
* Explain the parameters displayed on the ventilator panel
* Explain the relationship between oxygen saturation and alveolar ventilation

Monitoring is essential when you are looking after someone in acute respiratory failure, more so than when you are starting NIV electively in chronic hypercapnic respiratory failure.

Look at the patient

When you have started a patient on NIV, the most important thing to do is look at them from the bedside:

* Is their chest moving?
* Are they still using their accessory muscles?
* How comfortable do they look?

| Key Point | Terminology | Practical Tip | Physiology | How to do it |

Look at the patient first, then look at the ventilator: if the patient is not synchronising with the ventilator, then the numbers shown on the ventilator may be misleading.

Basic monitoring

The next thing to do when assessing how a patient is doing on NIV is to look at simple physiological variables:

- **Respiratory rate**
- **Pulse rate**
- **Blood pressure**
- **Oxygen saturation**

- **Respiratory rate**
  In many clinical situations a fast respiratory rate is an important indicator that the patient is very unwell. As they improve, the respiratory rate will gradually fall back to normal. This is true when NIV is used to treat acute respiratory failure, provided the patient is triggering the ventilator (as is usually the case with pressure-support, unless the back-up rate is set too high).

- **Pulse rate**
  Tachycardia is also common in acute respiratory failure, and a fall in pulse rate back towards normal when NIV is started is also a reassuring indicator that the patient is improving. Bradycardia is worrying, and implies an impending crisis (unless there is an obvious explanation such as beta-blockade).

- **Blood pressure**
  The blood pressure response to NIV is less predictable. If the patient is anxious or extremely unwell, they may be hypertensive initially, the blood pressure falling to more normal levels when they are settled on NIV. Conversely, the blood pressure may be low initially in a patient who is very hypoxic and hypercapnic, and may improve as NIV improves their gas exchange. NIV creates a positive pressure within the thorax, which may impair venous return to the heart and thus lower the blood pressure. This is uncommon, but you may need to reduce the IPAP and EPAP.

• **Oxygen saturation**

A patient with acute respiratory failure is likely to have their oxygen saturation monitored using a pulse oximeter and finger probe. This is extremely useful when the patient is breathing air. Aim for an SpO_2 of 88-92%. Much higher than this and you run the risk of suppressing the patient's own respiratory drive if there is any suggestion that respiratory failure is chronic.

If you struggle to get to 88%, this implies a serious problem with gas exchange in the lungs. You may then settle for a lower target range for oxygenation, say 85-90%.

Key Point	Terminology	Practical Tip	**Physiology**	How to do it

SpO_2 and hypercapnia when breathing supplementary oxygen
The alveolar air equation tells us about the partial pressure of oxygen in the alveoli. The abbreviation for this is PAO_2, with a capital A for alveolar:

$$PAO_2 = (FiO_2 \times 94) - (1.25 \times PaCO_2)$$

According to this equation, if the $PaCO_2$ rises, then PAO_2 must fall. If the patient is breathing air, they will desaturate and you will be alerted by an alarm on the oximeter.

PaO_2 is always slightly lower than PAO_2. Arterial oxygen desaturation below 90% occurs at PaO_2 around 8 kPa.

If the patient is breathing supplementary oxygen, the PAO_2 will remain high when the $PaCO_2$ rises, so an oximeter will not alert you to hypercapnia. The reason for this is apparent if you look at the first part of the equation: $FiO_2 \times 94$. Atmospheric pressure is 100 kPa, but we have to allow about 6 kPa to account for water vapour, since the alveolar air is fully humidified.

You may remember that FiO_2 is the fraction of inspired oxygen — 0.21 for air, which gives 20 for the first part of the equation (0.21 x 94). On 60% oxygen, this becomes 56 (0.60 x 94), so the $PaCO_2$ would have to rise to impossible levels before the PAO_2 fell to the levels associated with desaturation.

Blood gases

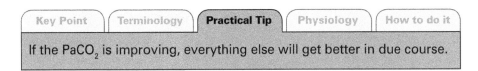

Key Point | Terminology | Practical Tip | Physiology | How to do it

If the patient is really sick, they need an arterial line.

You will need to check blood gases after about an hour of NIV, and an hour after any change in settings. If the patient is really sick and in ICU or HDU, you may choose to insert an arterial line. It takes a while for blood gas values to improve, and the $PaCO_2$ may lag behind the pH. Carbon dioxide tension can be monitored continuously using a transcutaneous electrode. The accuracy of the readings is improved if an arterial sample is taken initially to assess the arterial-transcutaneous difference. End-tidal carbon dioxide tensions (see Physiology) can be used to estimate $PaCO_2$, but should be used with caution in patients with abnormal lungs (i.e. most NIV patients).

Key Point | Terminology | **Practical Tip** | Physiology | How to do it

If the $PaCO_2$ is improving, everything else will get better in due course.

Key Point | Terminology | Practical Tip | **Physiology** | How to do it

End-tidal CO_2
If you have normal lungs, with fairly even matching of ventilation and perfusion, you can look at the concentration of CO_2 in the last bit of air you exhale to get an idea of what $PaCO_2$ is. Alveolar and arterial CO_2 levels are pretty similar, and the last bit of air you exhale will have come from deep down in your lungs, i.e. from the alveoli. This sample of air is called "end-tidal".

The problem with end-tidal CO_2 comes when the lungs have anything wrong with them. Some of the end-tidal gas will now come from areas of lung with little or no perfusion. This gas will look much like that which was inhaled, with no CO_2 in it. Mix this with the gas from normal lung and the end-tidal CO_2 is now much lower than in arterial blood (Figure 20.1).

cont ...

Key Point | Terminology | Practical Tip | **Physiology** | How to do it

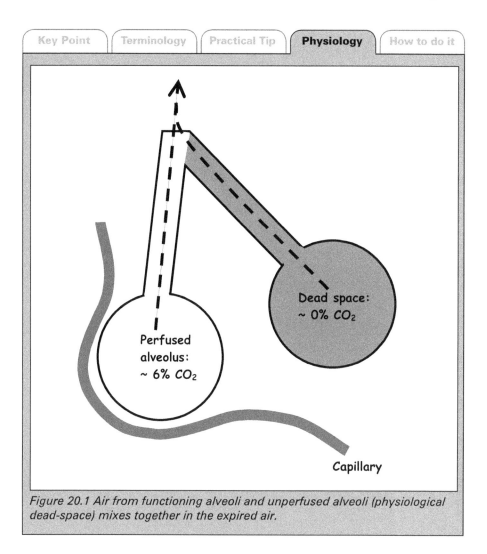

Figure 20.1 Air from functioning alveoli and unperfused alveoli (physiological dead-space) mixes together in the expired air.

The body's stores of oxygen are just over a litre, whereas there are over 100 litres of CO_2, when you take into account bicarbonate. As a result, any change in ventilation has a much more rapid effect on PaO_2 than $PaCO_2$.

Key Point | Terminology | **Practical Tip** | Physiology | How to do it

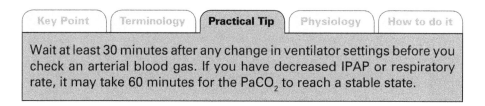

Wait at least 30 minutes after any change in ventilator settings before you check an arterial blood gas. If you have decreased IPAP or respiratory rate, it may take 60 minutes for the $PaCO_2$ to reach a stable state.

Watch out for a respiratory alkalosis when you lower $PaCO_2$ using NIV in a patient with chronic type 2 respiratory failure. The patient travels along their elevated bicarbonate line (as we saw in Figure 13.1 with acute-on-chronic hypercapnia), so the pH becomes alkalotic (Figure 20.2). (It would be difficult to work this out if we only saw one set of blood gas, not knowing how the patient got to that point.)

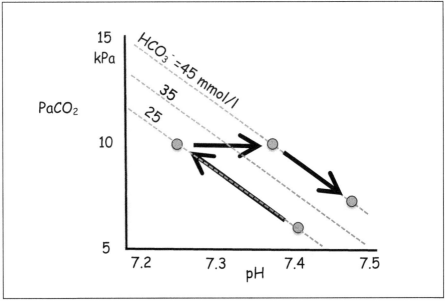

Figure 20.2 NIV will reduce $PaCO_2$. In a patient with chronic type 2 respiratory failure, this may result in a respiratory alkalosis. Even though the $PaCO_2$ is still greater than normal, it is lower than the steady state for that patient.

Other parameters

Of course, there are lots of other things you may choose to monitor in any individual, such as level of consciousness. The ventilator may generate parameters you are interested in charting — leak, compliance etc. Polysomnography is sometimes performed if it is particularly important to check if the patient is sleeping, for example when setting up NIV for long-term use at home.

The ventilator display

Some ventilators just have the control buttons and knobs on the front, but many have some sort of indicator to show how the ventilator is working. One simple version is a dial with a pointer which shows the pressure within the ventilator. This will swing between inspiration and expiration, in the way we have seen in the pressure-time traces earlier in this book (e.g. Figure 2.3). Another simple device is a bar which lights up to the height corresponding to pressure. With advances in computer technology, many modern ventilators have a graphical display. This might take the form of our pressure-time graph, often with flow at the same time. Add in a few icons to show you the mode of ventilation, some text with the back-up settings and current estimated Vt or minute ventilation and we have what — at first glance — is a pretty intimidating display. Don't panic. It is possible to use the display to help you straight away, even if it will take some time before you are fully conversant with every aspect. Look at the main trace of pressure and time; when you are happy, look at flow; then see how the flow is used to calculate volume, if this is included on the display. Start at one side of the display and look at each item in turn, making a note of those you don't understand. If you don't think you need to know about them at this stage, then leave them and visit them another time; if you think they might be important for you to know about at this stage, then ask someone or look in the manual.

Summary

- Look at the patient and the monitors
- Use an arterial line for sick patients
- Monitoring of respiratory rate, pulse, blood pressure and SpO_2 will suffice for less sick patients starting NIV in the acute setting

21
Alarms

Learning points

By the end of this chapter you should be able to:

- Decide what alarms you want to use
- Set low pressure and high flow alarms
- Explain how low pressure and high flow alarms detect disconnection
- Explain how low flow alarms detect occlusion

If you ask patients who have been on ICU, they think that every time an alarm goes off they are going to die. They cannot tell if it is their alarm or another patient's. Unlike the ICU staff, they cannot distinguish between a ventilator disconnection alarm and an infusion pump that has finished. This happens to a lesser extent with NIV, but it is still important to think about what you want an alarm to tell you about. Alarms often start to go off whilst you are setting a patient up on NIV. This is annoying, distracting and also undermines the patient's confidence in you. Use the option on the ventilator to silence the alarms until you have the patient settled on NIV.

Key Point	Terminology	Practical Tip	Physiology	How to do it

If an alarm is not going to be acted upon, it should be disabled.

Ventilator malfunction

If there is an internal problem with the ventilator, an alarm will usually go off. The ventilator will probably have stopped working, so the patient may well have taken off their mask already and alerted you to the problem. An alarm will sound if the ventilator becomes unplugged, or if the power fails. If the ventilator has an internal battery, a light may come on, and/or there may be an intermittent audible alarm to tell you that at some stage in the next few hours you need to get the power supply sorted out. Power alarms are often the only sensible alarms on a ventilator, in that they alert you to an important problem that you might not otherwise notice (i.e. that the ventilator has switched to its battery), they are usually acted on and are minimally intrusive to the clinical environment (often visible rather than audible).

Low pressure

Low pressure alarms have traditionally been the method used to detect a problem with the ventilator circuit. If you disconnect the circuit from a patient on NIV, the pressure-time trace will look like this (Figure 21.1):

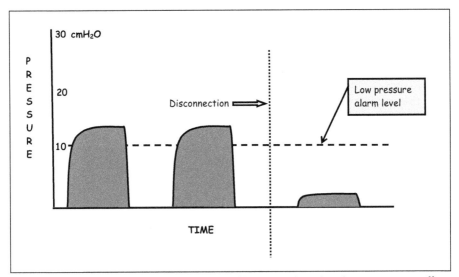

Figure 21.1 Low-pressure alarm to detect disconnection. An alarm set to go off if the pressure during inspiration doesn't get to 10 cmH$_2$O will detect this event. Notice how the pressure is not zero, because there is some resistance to flow in the circuit — if the alarm had been set to zero, it would not go off.

For ventilator-dependent patients, it may be advisable to have an independent low pressure alarm that is not integral to the ventilator, just in case the ventilator packs up and the internal alarms also stop working. These devices are more commonly used for patients ventilated through a tracheostomy. You could use an oxygen saturation monitor, but this means that you will only be alerted some time after ventilation has stopped and you will have even less time to sort things out.

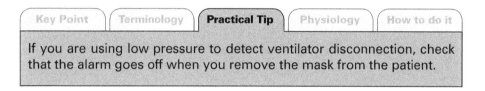

Key Point | Terminology | **Practical Tip** | Physiology | How to do it

If you are using low pressure to detect ventilator disconnection, check that the alarm goes off when you remove the mask from the patient.

High flow

If we add flow to this example, you can see how the flow delivered by the ventilator shoots up when the disconnection occurs, as the ventilator tries to get the pressure up to the target IPAP (Figure 21.2):

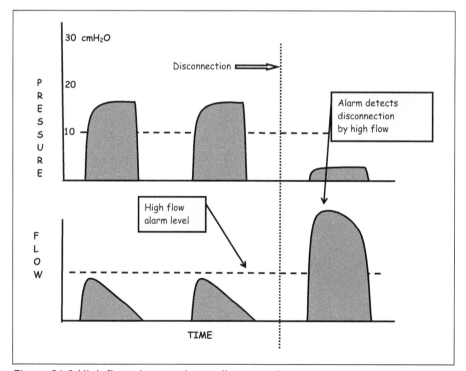

Figure 21.2 High-flow alarm to detect disconnection.

Many modern NIV ventilators use high flow alarms to detect disconnection. Measuring flow also allows you to notice when a mask develops a leak, because there is an increase in flow, even if there isn't much change in the pressure.

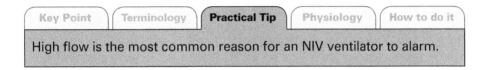

Key Point	Terminology	**Practical Tip**	Physiology	How to do it

High flow is the most common reason for an NIV ventilator to alarm.

Low flow

If the ventilator circuit is occluded, for example if secretions have clogged up a filter, then the target pressure will be reached with very little flow from the ventilator. Low flow alarms can also alert you to occlusion of the upper airway, again because the target pressure is reached too easily (Figure 21.3):

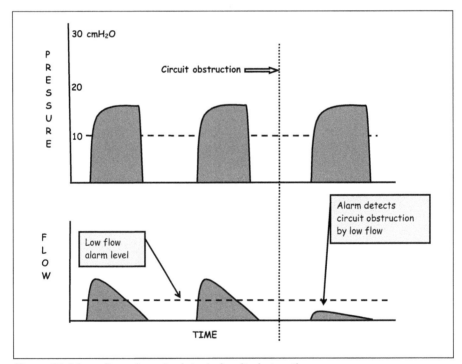

Figure 21.3 Low-flow alarm to detect circuit obstruction.

High pressure

During ventilation through an endotracheal tube, a high pressure alarm is needed to alert you if excessively high pressures are being applied to the lung. With NIV, high pressures just blow the mask off the face, so a high pressure alarm is redundant.

In volume-controlled ventilation (see Chapter 40) a set volume is delivered; if the patient's condition deteriorates or the circuit becomes occluded, an alarm may be used to alert you to the excessively high pressures which are needed to maintain tidal volume.

Tidal volume and minute ventilation

Most modern NIV ventilators also estimate volume from the amount of air they have had to blow in to the patient.

A much more accurate assessment of volume can be made by incorporating a flow-measuring device into the circuit near the mask. Vt is estimated by these devices during expiration, to get over the problem that some of the inspiratory flow will have been wasted on leaks around the mask.

As we saw earlier, adding all the breaths in a minute gives you minute ventilation. Alarm thresholds for this can also be set.

Remote alarms

An alarm needs to alert someone to do something about the condition which has set it off. This might be a carer elsewhere in the house, so the alarm needs to be very loud. Some ventilators will allow you to connect a remote loudspeaker using a long cable. Environmental control engineers will be able to help connect the ventilator to a remote alarm.

Summary

- Alarms have a tendency to be more of a hindrance than a help
- Keep it simple — use as few alarms as you can
- A high flow alarm is probably the most useful — use it to tell you if the mask has become disconnected or dislodged

22
Left Ventricular Failure

Learning points

By the end of this chapter you should be able to:

- Decide which patients with acute LVF need NIV
- Set a patient with LVF up on NIV
- Say what to look for to make sure that NIV is working
- Decide where to manage a patient with LVF on NIV
- Discuss the use of NIV in chronic heart failure

Sometimes it can be difficult to decide whether acute breathlessness is COPD or LVF. The good news is that NIV works for both, although there has been quite a lot of debate about its use in heart failure. Some early trials used NIV without much else in the way of drug treatment, and in one of the first randomised studies the cohort of patients who were treated with NIV, by chance, had more severe myocardial ischaemia and not surprisingly did less well.

NIV or CPAP

Subsequent larger trials have shown that NIV and CPAP are equally effective in improving the physiology of patients with acute LVF. The advantage of CPAP is that it is easier to set up, and you don't have to worry about triggering and synchronisation. These patients are often pretty tachypnoeic, and they tend to settle onto CPAP better than NIV.

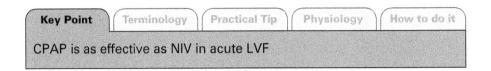

Key Point	Terminology	Practical Tip	Physiology	How to do it

CPAP is as effective as NIV in acute LVF

If the patient is hypercapnic and this doesn't improve within an hour on CPAP, you could switch to NIV. You may also choose to start with NIV if it is more readily available than CPAP.

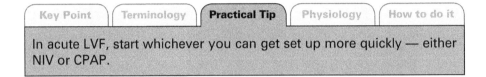

Key Point	Terminology	Practical Tip	Physiology	How to do it

In acute LVF, start whichever you can get set up more quickly — either NIV or CPAP.

Ventilator settings

Use bi-level pressure-support starting with an IPAP of 10 cmH$_2$O and an EPAP of 5 cmH$_2$O. Depending on the patient's respiratory pattern, this is equivalent to using CPAP of about 7.5 cmH$_2$O, which would be quite a reasonable starting level if we weren't using NIV.

Nudge both the IPAP and EPAP down 2 cmH$_2$O if the patient's blood pressure does drop.

Increasing the IPAP to 15 cmH$_2$O will help a persistently elevated PaCO$_2$, whereas increasing the EPAP to 7 or 8 cmH$_2$O should improve oxygenation.

Set the back-up rate to about 12 breaths/min, with an inspiratory:expiratory ratio of 1:2.

Where?

Start NIV or CPAP early in LVF — you don't have as much time to play with as in COPD. The patient will need ECG and saturation monitoring, so they really need to be on a coronary care unit, HDU or ICU as soon as possible. The decision between CCU and HDU will depend on whether other cardiac therapy (such as thrombolysis) is needed, how likely serious cardiac dysrhythmias are and the NIV experience of CCU staff.

How long for?

A few hours is often all that is necessary. After this time, drug therapy will have kicked in and the patient will start to improve.

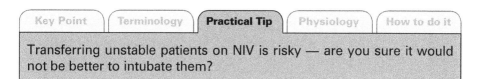

Key Point | Terminology | Practical Tip | Physiology | **How to do it**

Transfer a patient on NIV
- Check that the receiving clinical area is ready
- Things tend to become dislodged during transfer — ensure all vascular lines, the NIV mask etc. are secured in place
- If the NIV ventilator does not have an internal battery, connect an external one
- Check that the batteries are fully charged
- If the patient needs supplementary oxygen, change the supply to a cylinder
- Secure the ventilator, battery and oxygen cylinder to the trolley or bed, in a position where they cannot fall onto the floor or onto the patient
- Attach a battery-powered pulse oximeter to the patient
- Position the oximeter display so that you can see it all the time during the transfer
- Take a resuscitation bag and mask with you
- If the patient would be for intubation if they deteriorate, take the appropriate equipment with you
- Transfer the patient

Most patients on NIV can manage spontaneous breathing for a few minutes: it is much easier to transfer a patient off NIV.

Key Point | Terminology | **Practical Tip** | Physiology | How to do it

Transferring unstable patients on NIV is risky — are you sure it would not be better to intubate them?

Cheyne-Stokes respiration
Some patients with chronic heart failure have disturbed sleep, usually associated with Cheyne-Stoke's respiration (CSR). This is a cyclical increase and decrease in Vt, so that sometimes the patient is hyperventilating and sometimes they stop breathing (Figure 22.1).

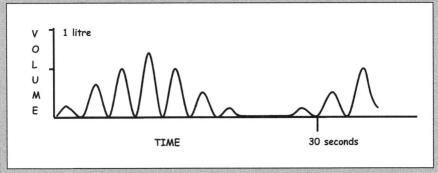

Figure 22.1 A cycle of CSR is a slow decrease in Vt, a brief apnoea, then a gradual increase in Vt again. A cycle takes about 30 seconds or so.

There are all sorts of theories about the aetiology of CSR in heart failure. Most of these patients are slightly hypocapnic, perhaps because vasculature congestion stimulates lung receptors to increase ventilation. Hypocapnia tends to stop you breathing, so ventilatory control becomes unstable. The feedback loop to correct underventilation or overventilation may also be too slow, as a result of poor cardiac output and hence longer circulation time.

It seems that most of the adverse effects on the patient of CSR come from the arousal from sleep which is common in the hyperventilation phase of this pattern of breathing. There is a burst of sympathetic activity associated with the arousal.

NIV in chronic heart failure

We are still exploring the role of nocturnal NIV in chronic heart failure — the number of patients who benefit is likely to remain small, given that excessive daytime sleepiness (in contrast to fatigue) is an uncommon symptom in this condition. Oxygen therapy is quite effective, and is much easier for the patient than NIV. Reducing the degree of hypoxia with each cycle of apnoea will prevent many of the arousals from sleep.

If you do decide on a therapeutic trial, be clear about what you are trying to achieve. Re-assess after an appropriate interval and discontinue NIV if your goal has not been achieved. This goal will usually be better quality sleep, but might also be improvement in heart failure.

Use bi-level pressure-support, with similar settings to those we chose for acute LVF. We'll look at volume-controlled ventilation in more detail later. It is possible to use a ventilator which will follow the cyclical changes in Vt of CSR. Patients tend to find this more comfortable than conventional NIV.

Key Point	Terminology	Practical Tip	Physiology	How to do it

Nocturnal supplementary oxygen is better than NIV for most patients with chronic heart failure.

Key Point	Terminology	Practical Tip	**Physiology**	How to do it

Oxygen delivery
We have talked already about PaO_2 and SpO_2. Remember that the oxygen content of blood is also dependent on the haemoglobin concentration: the number of millilitres of oxygen in each litre is given by the following equation:

$$SpO_2 \times Hb \times 1.34 \text{ (with Hb in g/l)}$$

The blood also needs to be transported to the peripheral tissues, so clearly cardiac output will be important. Cardiac output depends on the volume of blood leaving the heart with each beat (stroke volume) and the heart rate. Oxygen delivery can be calculated by:

$$\text{Stroke volume} \times \text{heart rate} \times SpO_2 \times Hb \times 1.34$$

The 1.34 value isn't important to remember, but bear the other factors in mind when you are trying to maximise oxygen delivery to the peripheral tissues in a patient with heart failure.

Summary

- CPAP is an effective treatment for LVF
- Use it if the patient does not respond to initial drug therapy
- If you use NIV, keep the pressures fairly low
- Don't forget to give drugs
- Stop NIV as soon as the patient is better

23
Sleep

Learning points

By the end of this chapter you should be able to:

- Outline the changes to breathing that occur during the different phases of sleep
- Explain why rapid-eye-movement sleep is a particularly vulnerable time for patients with respiratory problems

Many of our patients will only use NIV at night. It is less intrusive to have a mask on whilst you are asleep. Might using NIV at night just be a matter of convenience, much like putting your mobile phone on charge overnight?

This doesn't seem to be the case for most patients. Sleep is a particularly bad time for them, and they need NIV to allow them to sleep properly. Let's have a look at what happens during sleep and see if we can work out why NIV has such a beneficial effect.

Ventilation

During deep sleep, our brains are busy sifting through information and deciding what to do with it. General "automatic" background brain activity is all slightly reduced during sleep. This applies to ventilation as much as anything else. Our bodies are much less active than during the daytime, so we don't need as much ventilation anyway.

Respiratory drive

Respiratory drive is reduced during sleep. This applies to hypoxic and hypercapnic drive and reflects the general reduction in the brain's responsiveness.

Muscle tone

Muscle tone is reduced during sleep. For the respiratory muscles, they produce less force for any given neural drive to them.

For the upper airways, reduction in pharyngeal muscle tone causes an increase in upper airway resistance. This also reduces the amount of ventilation generated for a set amount of inspiratory muscle contraction.

A decrease in intercostal muscle tone, particularly during REM sleep (see below), means that the volume of the lungs is reduced. As a consequence, there is less oxygen stored in the lungs to act as a buffer during apnoeas (see next section).

Key Point	Terminology	Practical Tip	**Physiology**	How to do it

Lung volume and oxygen stores

If you stop breathing at the end of a tidal breath — i.e. at functional residual capacity (FRC) — there will be about 3 litres of air still in your lungs; 15% of this is oxygen, about 450 ml.

Oxygen consumption at rest is about 200 ml/min, so you'll run out of oxygen in about 2 minutes.

For a patient with a restrictive ventilatory defect, FRC may only be 500ml or so; 15% of this is only 75 ml — enough to last less than 30 seconds.

Low intra-pulmonary oxygen stores probably contribute to the severity of hypoxaemia seen in diseases such as scoliosis and neuromuscular disease.

Rapid-eye-movement sleep

Sleep is divided into different stages. Traditionally, a sleep study is cut up into "epochs" of thirty seconds, to each of which is assigned a "stage" according to rules published by Rechstaffen and Kales (known as R & K in the trade) in 1968. Stages 1 and 2 are light sleep; stages 3 and 4 are deep "restorative" sleep. Another stage of sleep is known as "rapid-eye-movement" or REM sleep (Figure 23.1).

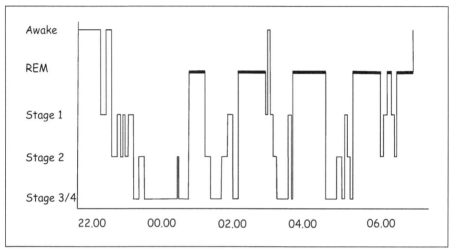

Figure 23.1 Overnight hypnogram, showing the time spent in different stages of sleep.

There does seem to be something very different about REM sleep. REM sleep is about dreaming. To stop you from acting out your dreams, your limb muscles become paralysed. The only respiratory muscle which keeps working is the diaphragm. The intercostal, abdominal and accessory muscles are all treated as limb muscles and are paralysed during REM sleep.

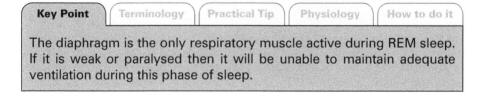

Key Point | Terminology | Practical Tip | Physiology | How to do it

The diaphragm is the only respiratory muscle active during REM sleep. If it is weak or paralysed then it will be unable to maintain adequate ventilation during this phase of sleep.

We noted in Chapter 7 that $PaCO_2$ was higher during sleep than the daytime. It is higher still during REM sleep (Figure 23.2). Ventilation is much more irregular in REM sleep.

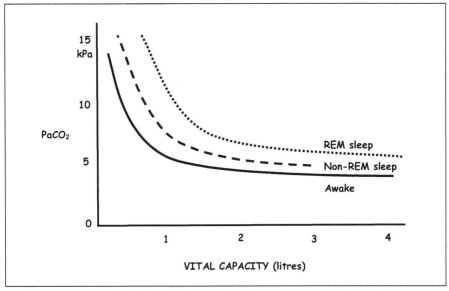

Figure 23.2 $PaCO_2$ is highest during REM sleep.

Symptoms of hypoventilation during sleep

Classically, patients with nocturnal hypoventilation wake up during the night feeling short of breath and have a headache in the morning. The headache is caused by hypercapnia and may be present during the night as well. More commonly patients will just feel that they haven't slept well and are unrefreshed in the morning. Witnesses will often say that they are very restless sleepers. Hypoxia during sleep causes a diuresis, so ask about nocturia.

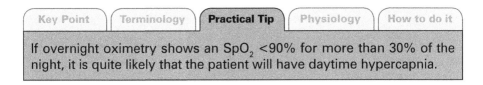

Key Point | Terminology | **Practical Tip** | Physiology | How to do it

If overnight oximetry shows an SpO_2 <90% for more than 30% of the night, it is quite likely that the patient will have daytime hypercapnia.

The net result of poor sleep is sleepiness during the daytime. This pathological daytime sleepiness is more debilitating than just feeling tired. Ask about situations where your patient has fallen asleep against their will — going to sleep during meals or conversations is more worrying than just nodding off in front of the television after an evening meal.

Some patients whose sleep study shows significant nocturnal hypoventilation have absolutely no symptoms. A few feel better if you start them on nocturnal NIV, having forgotten what it feels like to have a normal night's sleep, but there are others who are genuinely asymptomatic. If they are at risk of running into trouble, for example if they have a progressive neuromuscular condition, be wary of asking them just to come back and see you if they develop symptoms — the onset of symptoms is very gradual and they may not notice until they have a crisis.

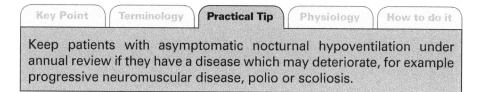

Key Point | Terminology | **Practical Tip** | Physiology | How to do it

Keep patients with asymptomatic nocturnal hypoventilation under annual review if they have a disease which may deteriorate, for example progressive neuromuscular disease, polio or scoliosis.

Daytime arterial blood gases

If the daytime $PaCO_2$ is elevated, it is highly likely to be even higher at night. For many such patients a sleep study isn't really necessary. Just start NIV.

Keep a close eye on the bicarbonate level. If $PaCO_2$ is up at night for any length of time, the bicarbonate will be elevated.

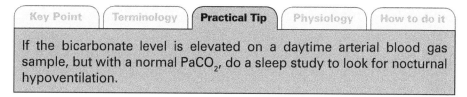

Key Point | Terminology | **Practical Tip** | Physiology | How to do it

If the bicarbonate level is elevated on a daytime arterial blood gas sample, but with a normal $PaCO_2$, do a sleep study to look for nocturnal hypoventilation.

Some people like to do an "early morning" blood gas, on the pretext that you will catch $PaCO_2$ whilst it is still up. I don't find it particularly helpful. Better to do a sleep study.

Sleep studies

There is a hierarchy of sleep studies.

- **Oximetry**
  This is simple and cheap. If results are completely normal, significant hypoventilation is unlikely (provided the patient is not breathing supplementary oxygen during the study).

- **Transcutaneous capnography**
  We've talked about CO_2 as the most crucial variable in deciding when to use NIV. Transcutaneous CO_2 monitors are great for seeing if patients underventilate at night, and particularly useful if you want to confirm that NIV is providing effective ventilation. They are much more cumbersome and expensive than oximeters, though.

- **Limited-channel sleep studies**
  This is oximetry, but with measurements of airflow, sound, chest wall movement, position etc.

- **Polysomnography**
  Add in EEG and you get full polysomnography. The advantages are that you can be sure your patient slept during the study, and see if any respiratory events woke them up. It is a time consuming and expensive method but the only way of telling for sure whether the patient is asleep or not, which stage of sleep they are in and whether any ventilation-related events wake them up from sleep.

Summary

- **Sleep is a bad time for many respiratory patients**
- **REM sleep is particularly bad**

24
Expiratory Pressure

Learning points

By the end of this chapter you should be able to:

- Define EPAP
- Set the upper and lower limits you would normally use for EPAP
- List the physiological effects of EPAP
- Discuss the clinical situations in which it may be helpful to alter EPAP

For most patients on bi-level ventilation, an EPAP of 5 cmH$_2$O will be fine. You don't need to adjust it very often. IPAP is much more important. As you become more conversant with NIV you may start to adjust the EPAP from time to time, but the range is pretty narrow and the benefits usually small. Many patients find EPAP a bit uncomfortable, and few will tolerate more than 10 cmH$_2$O.

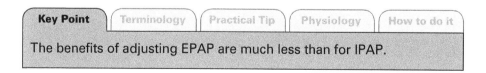

Key Point | Terminology | Practical Tip | Physiology | How to do it

The benefits of adjusting EPAP are much less than for IPAP.

Flushing CO_2 out of the circuit

We have seen how EPAP flushes exhaled air out of the expiratory port of the circuit, allowing us to use a single tube. If the patient settles well onto NIV and their chest seems to be expanding well in time with the ventilation but the $PaCO_2$ fails to fall, it is worth just thinking about increasing the EPAP a little in case re-breathing is occurring. The higher the EPAP the more flow there will be out of the expiratory port. Remember that increasing the EPAP will also flush oxygen out of the circuit. If you have a single-tube bi-level circuit, don't reduce EPAP below 3 cmH$_2$O.

Upper airway patency

EPAP keeps the upper airway open, just as CPAP does in the treatment of obstructive sleep apnoea. Although IPAP would open the airway in due course anyway, the fact that it is held open by EPAP allows the ventilator to sense when the patient wants to take the next breath in. If a very obese patient appears to be trying to take a breath in, but the ventilator is not triggering, think about upper airway obstruction — try increasing the EPAP. We'll come back to this when we talk about the obesity-hypoventilation syndrome in Chapter 28.

Oxygenation

EPAP increases lung volume, which is good if there is a problem with oxygenation on account of lung collapse (atelectasis) in the lower parts of the lung. There is a down side to increasing lung volume, in that you may over-inflate the more distensible parts of the lung. The blood vessels in over-inflated areas of lung are stretched and thin, so you may divert blood towards the stiffer parts of the lung which can't over-inflate — these may well be areas of diseased lung which don't exchange gas very well.

Ventilation

In type 1 respiratory failure, we may choose to use an EPAP of up to 10 cmH$_2$O. You may remember from the chapter on IPAP that this reduces the difference between IPAP and EPAP, so the tidal volume will be less — keep an eye on the $PaCO_2$.

Over-inflation is particularly bad for COPD patients, putting their respiratory muscles at even more of a mechanical disadvantage than they are already.

Cardiac output

EPAP increases the pressure inside the chest, and this may impede the return of venous blood from the periphery — if the mean intra-thoracic pressure is high, the pressure needed to push the blood back into the heart is higher. The result of this is that cardiac output may fall. If there is a fall in blood pressure on BIPAP, reduce both the IPAP and EPAP and consider administering intravenous fluids.

Intrinsic PEEP

Intrinsic PEEP (PEEPi or "autopeep" as it is sometimes called) is a particular feature of patients with airflow obstruction such as COPD. It is a difficult concept to explain, not made any easier by the difficulty of measuring it — you would need an oesophageal pressure probe or balloon.

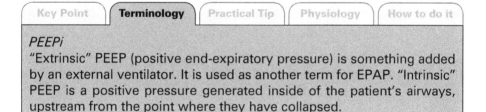

Key Point	Terminology	Practical Tip	Physiology	How to do it

PEEPi
"Extrinsic" PEEP (positive end-expiratory pressure) is something added by an external ventilator. It is used as another term for EPAP. "Intrinsic" PEEP is a positive pressure generated inside of the patient's airways, upstream from the point where they have collapsed.

So, let's ignore the "PEEP" bit, forget about the "intrinsic" bit and concentrate on why PEEPi makes it hard work for COPD patients to trigger inspiration during NIV.

If you take a breath in and then relax all your respiratory and upper airway muscles, the air in your lungs flows out quickly, usually much less than one second. When you contract your inspiratory muscles, inward airflow starts straight away, and if you were connected to an NIV ventilator, inspiration would be triggered immediately.

In a patient with narrow airways, it could take up to 30 seconds for the lungs to empty completely. Clearly a patient with COPD is not going to take one breath every minute, they cannot breathe that slowly, so the result is that they have not fully exhaled when they start to take the next breath in (Figure 24.1).

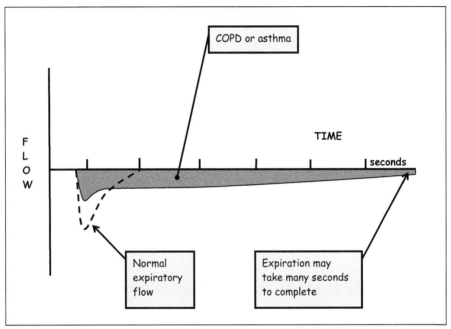

Figure 24.1 Expiratory flow persists for many seconds if you disconnect an intubated patient with COPD or asthma from the ventilator.

Let's suppose that there is still a litre of air in the lungs left to exhale when they have to take another breath in. The inspiratory muscles have to contract as if they were inhaling this litre before they get to the position where the lungs have stopped because of the trapped air. Only then does flow start and trigger the ventilator. The pressure that the inspiratory muscles have to generate before there is any airflow is equivalent to PEEPi (Figure 24.2).

You can use EPAP to help the patient overcome PEEPi. Increasing the EPAP means that the patient will start from a point much nearer the lung volume they are trapped at, so they don't need to make such a big effort to get some flow and trigger the ventilator (Figure 24.2):

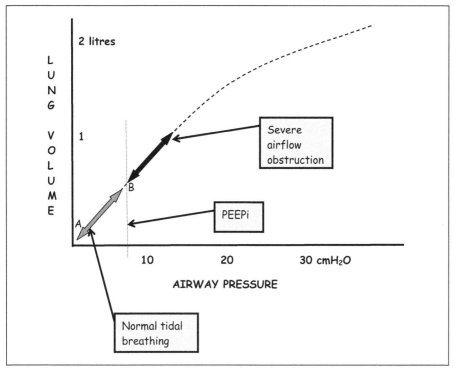

Figure 24.2 Intrinsic PEEP. At the end of expiration, someone with normal lungs would be at point A; when they generate pressure to inflate their lungs, by using their inspiratory muscles, volume starts to increase straight away — if they were on NIV, this change in volume (flow) would be sensed by the ventilator which would immediately assist the breath. In severe COPD, airway collapse means that at the end of expiration the patient has so much air trapped in their lung that they are at point B; when they contract their inspiratory muscles, there will be no change in lung volume until they have generated a pressure equivalent to being at point B — only then is there any flow to tell the ventilator that they want to take a breath in.

IPAP profile

One final point about EPAP: With an expiratory valve, there is an abrupt change from IPAP to zero pressure. Once the valve is open, there is a rapid fall in pressure over which we have no control. Patients don't usually mind this too much.

With bi-level ventilation we can ask the ventilator to switch from IPAP to EPAP as slowly or quickly as we like. This gives us the opportunity to set a more gentle transition from inspiration to expiration, which can be more comfortable (Figure 24.3).

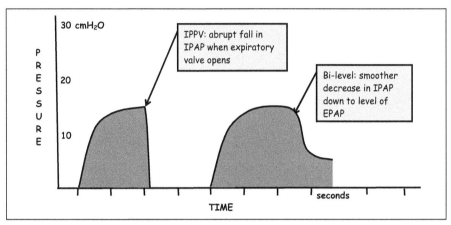

Figure 24.3 EPAP allows a more gradual end to inspiration.

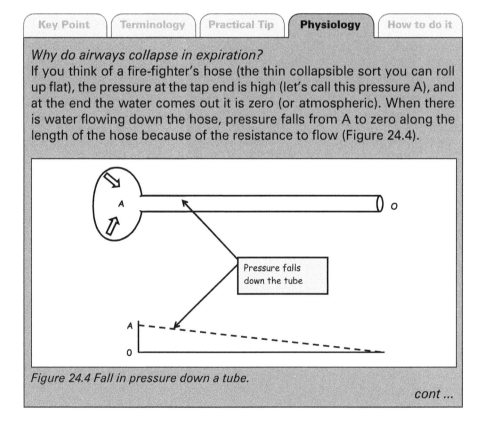

Why do airways collapse in expiration?
If you think of a fire-fighter's hose (the thin collapsible sort you can roll up flat), the pressure at the tap end is high (let's call this pressure A), and at the end the water comes out it is zero (or atmospheric). When there is water flowing down the hose, pressure falls from A to zero along the length of the hose because of the resistance to flow (Figure 24.4).

Figure 24.4 Fall in pressure down a tube.

cont ...

Key Point | Terminology | Practical Tip | **Physiology** | How to do it

Imagine putting the tap and the hose inside a big tank, leaving the end of the hose sticking out, and pressurising the tank — let's call this pressure B. The "driving pressure" at the tap end of the hose is now the tap pressure plus the pressure inside the tank. The pressure at the hose outlet is still zero, so the pressure inside the hose must fall steadily from A+B to zero as we move from the tap to the open end. The pressure outside the hose is B all the way along its length, because it is inside the tank. At some point along the length of the hose, as pressure falls from A+B to zero, this pressure will become less than B and the hose will collapse (Figure 24.5).

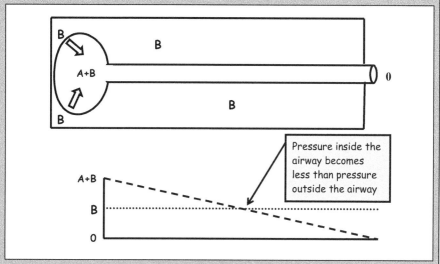

Figure 24.5 Fall in pressure down the tube when surrounded by a positive pressure.

In the lungs, A is the elastic recoil of the alveoli and B is the expiratory pressure we generate with our expiratory muscles. Usually A is sufficiently high that the pressure inside the hose doesn't fall from A+B to B until we reach the large airways, which are splinted open by cartilage and don't collapse. If A is very low, because of emphysema, then the pressure inside the airways falls to B very quickly and the airways collapse (Figure 24.6).

cont ...

Key Point | Terminology | Practical Tip | **Physiology** | How to do it

This leads us to another way to think about PEEPi, using the collapsing tube model of airflow obstruction. When the airway collapses at the "equal pressure point", there is no flow in the patent bit of the airway which is therefore all at the same pressure. This is the elastic recoil pressure, which we called "A" previously. This is exactly the same pressure we are now referring to as PEEPi.

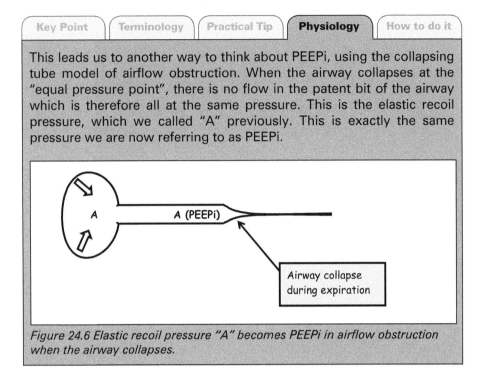

Figure 24.6 Elastic recoil pressure "A" becomes PEEPi in airflow obstruction when the airway collapses.

Summary

- **EPAP flushes CO_2 out of bi-level circuits**
- **Upper airway patency is maintained**
- **Lung volume is increased**
- **Cardiac output may decrease**
- **EPAP helps overcome PEEPi**

25
Central Sleep Apnoea

Learning points

By the end of this chapter you should be able to:

* Describe how central sleep apnoea differs from obstructive sleep apnoea
* Give some examples of disease processes that cause central sleep apnoea

Every long-term NIV service has a small group of patients with central sleep apnoea. If you exclude those with obesity-hypoventilation (Chapter 28) and heart failure (Chapter 22), the rest are something of a mixed bag. The unifying factor is that they stop breathing at night and usually get much better when you start them on NIV.

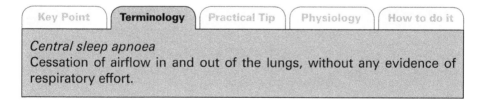

| Key Point | **Terminology** | Practical Tip | Physiology | How to do it |

Central sleep apnoea
Cessation of airflow in and out of the lungs, without any evidence of respiratory effort.

Aetiology

Central hypoventilation is a common reason for starting NIV in children. Some have a neurological diagnosis such as dysautonomia where it is not unexpected that there is a problem with regulation of breathing. Others have a neurological problem where it seems plausible that the pathology has involved the cerebral respiratory centres. A few have nothing else wrong with them apart from central sleep apnoea, reflecting a congenital deficiency of function in the brainstem respiratory centres. The genetics underlying such defects is gradually becoming clearer.

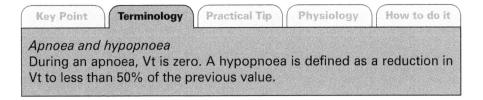

| Key Point | **Terminology** | Practical Tip | Physiology | How to do it |

Apnoea and hypopnoea
During an apnoea, Vt is zero. A hypopnoea is defined as a reduction in Vt to less than 50% of the previous value.

In adults, a few patients with central sleep apnoea have other neurological diagnoses. These include:

- **Stroke**
- **Arterio-venous malformation**
- **Demyelination**
- **Inflammation**
- **Poliomyelitis**
- **Encephalitis**
- **Trauma**
- **Surgery**

Most don't have any clinical evidence of neurological disease, and it is very unusual to find anything if you image their brains. Whilst it seems prudent to keep looking for the development of other neurological problems, this doesn't usually happen.

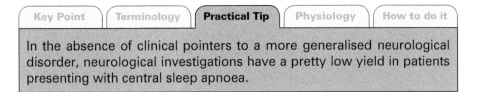

| Key Point | Terminology | **Practical Tip** | Physiology | How to do it |

In the absence of clinical pointers to a more generalised neurological disorder, neurological investigations have a pretty low yield in patients presenting with central sleep apnoea.

Cervical cord lesions

Curiously, central sleep apnoea is seen in some patients with cervical cord problems such as Arnold-Chiari malformations. The reasons for this are not clear. Perhaps disruption of the neuronal links between the cord and the respiratory centres destabilises respiratory control.

Upper airway obstruction

Obstruction of the upper airway, either due to pharyngeal collapse or laryngospasm, can induce reflex central apnoea. This can be quite difficult to sort out on a sleep study. Is the central component of a mixed central and obstructive apnoea the consequence of obesity-hypoventilation; is it reflexive from the obstruction; or is it poor central drive because of chronic sleep deprivation?

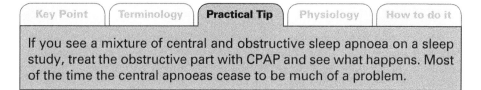

| Key Point | Terminology | **Practical Tip** | Physiology | How to do it |

If you see a mixture of central and obstructive sleep apnoea on a sleep study, treat the obstructive part with CPAP and see what happens. Most of the time the central apnoeas cease to be much of a problem.

NIV

For central sleep apnoea, use IPPV. Bi-level pressure-control would be my next choice. If the main problem is central drive, without any associated obesity or chest wall deformity, then an IPAP of 15 cmH$_2$O will be sufficient. Overnight monitoring of CO$_2$ is important to check that ventilation is adequate, but also to ensure that you don't hyperventilate the patient.

Laryngeal obstruction and NIV

When your patient stops breathing during sleep, their vocal cords rest together and close off the airway. We probably all do this when we have brief apnoeas during REM sleep, but it doesn't give us a problem because we're not trying to get air through our cords and into the lungs. It is a problem if you are using NIV. If you watch a patient asleep whilst on NIV, there will be times when their chest doesn't move. This implies that there is something preventing IPAP from reaching the lungs and inflating them. If the obstruction is laryngeal there's not much you can do about it — increasing EPAP won't do anything. NIV does seem to help, maybe by increasing the size of breaths as soon as the cords open a little. Tracheostomy is sometimes the only option.

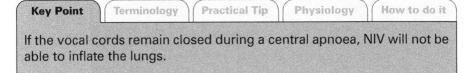

Key Point | Terminology | Practical Tip | Physiology | How to do it

If the vocal cords remain closed during a central apnoea, NIV will not be able to inflate the lungs.

Key Point | Terminology | Practical Tip | **Physiology** | How to do it

Respiratory drive
You can measure respiratory drive by filling a large bag (20 litres or so) with oxygen and breathing in and out of it for a few minutes. There will be sufficient oxygen to prevent your SpO_2 dropping, but CO_2 will build up in the bag. As you start to re-breathe this CO_2, your $PaCO_2$ will rise. This will stimulate your respiratory centre and make you breathe deeper and faster. You can measure the slope of the increase in ventilation as CO_2 rises. If your respiratory drive is poor, you will see a much smaller increase in ventilation (Figure 25.1).

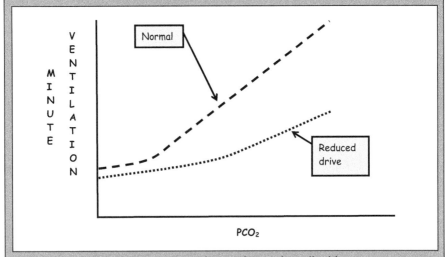

Figure 25.1 Ventilatory response to increasing carbon dioxide.

cont ...

| Key Point | Terminology | Practical Tip | **Physiology** | How to do it |

Hypercapnia is a more important factor than hypoxia in driving respiration. However, in chronic type 2 respiratory failure, the respiratory centre gets used to a high CO_2 (and any increase in CO_2 is buffered by the large "pool" of bicarbonate) — and hypoxic drive becomes more important. Abolishing hypoxic drive — by administering supplementary oxygen — will reduce ventilation even further.

The increase in ventilation depends not only on respiratory drive, but also on how easy it is to get air in and out of the lungs. One way of overcoming this difficulty is to block off the mouthpiece — without the patient knowing — and measure the pressure 0.1 seconds after they start trying to take a breath in. This is called the P0.1 value. In practice, measuring respiratory drive is quite difficult. As with so many of the more sophisticated tests of lung function, the normal ranges are not well defined.

| Key Point | Terminology | **Practical Tip** | Physiology | How to do it |

Use acetazolamide for a few days in patients with nocturnal hypoventilation and bicarbonate levels >35 mmol/l, whilst you get on top of their $PaCO_2$. This will reduce their bicarbonate pool and increase their responsiveness to CO_2.

Summary

- Central sleep apnoea is much less common than obstructive sleep apnoea
- The cause isn't usually apparent
- It responds to NIV, provided the patient's vocal cords remain open during the apnoea

26
Triggering

Learning points

By the end of this chapter you should be able to:

• Describe how a patient can trigger a breath in
• Describe how a pressure-support ventilator decides when to switch from inspiration to expiration
• Know when to adjust trigger sensitivity
• Define autotriggering

Triggering inspiration

All NIV ventilators will allow the patient to trigger the start of the next breath. In older ventilators this involves pressure triggering, where the patient has to generate a small negative pressure to tell the ventilator that they want to take a breath in. Most modern ventilators use flow triggers: when the ventilator detects a small inspiratory flow, this then activates inspiratory pressure generation (Figure 26.1).

173

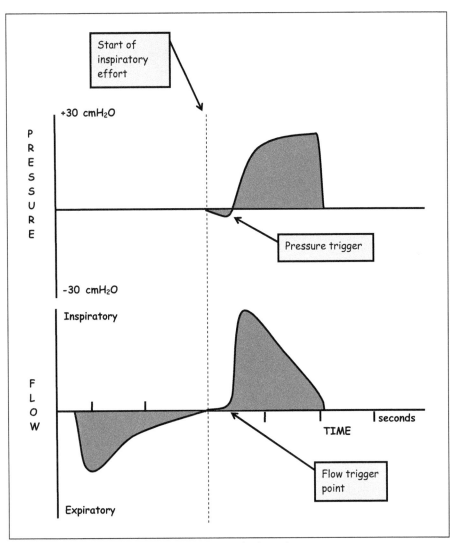

Figure 26.1 Pressure and flow at the start of a breath.

There is a "window" during which it is possible for the patient to trigger a breath. The ventilator won't allow them to do it too early, otherwise there wouldn't be enough time to exhale the previous breath. Too late and the back-up rate kicks in (Figure 26.2).

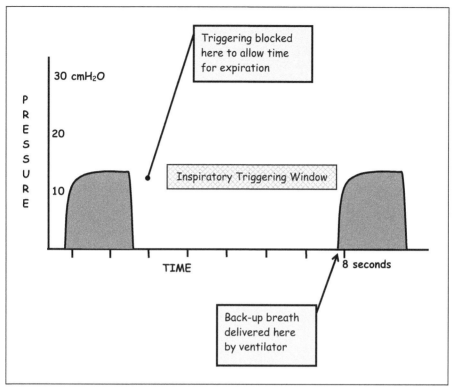

Figure 26.2 The window during which a patient can trigger inspiration.

If you have a patient who is struggling to co-ordinate their breathing with the ventilator, you can try a more sensitive inspiratory trigger. Watch the patient breathing on the ventilator to make sure you haven't made the trigger so sensitive that it is triggering even when the patient isn't trying to breathe in.

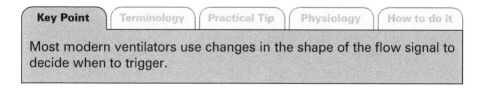

Key Point	Terminology	Practical Tip	Physiology	How to do it

Most modern ventilators use changes in the shape of the flow signal to decide when to trigger.

Triggering expiration

With pressure-control, expiration is not triggered but occurs after a set amount of time. You choose this time, not the patient. Having watched the patient breathing spontaneously, you might choose an inspiratory time of 1.5 seconds and set the ventilator accordingly.

For bi-level pressure-support we have seen how the patient triggers the ventilator across from inspiration to expiration (Figure 8.2). Again this is best done by detecting a fall in flow rate — at the end of a breath in, there is less and less air entering the lungs, and when flow falls below a set level then it is time to withdraw the IPAP and change to expiration.

In patients with COPD the peak expiratory flow may be very low, and it may take too long to reach 30% of this level. Increasing the cut-off to 50%, or even 70%, of maximum flow will be more comfortable for the patient — the flow levels may not be specified, but just marked as "sensitivity". Shortening inspiration will allow them more time to breathe out and reduce the chances of them becoming over-inflated. Watch carefully to check that they get a reasonable breath in, and don't switch across to expiration too early (Figure 26.3).

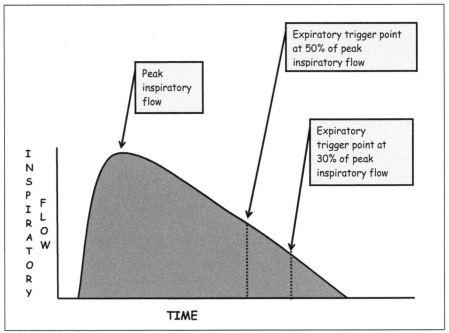

Figure 26.3 Changing the expiratory trigger level to 50% of peak inspiratory flow will shorten the duration of inspiration.

There is always a maximum time set for inspiration, irrespective of what is happening to flow. This is a safety mechanism, so that the ventilator doesn't blow for thirty seconds whilst waiting for flow to reach a particular trigger level (Figure 26.4).

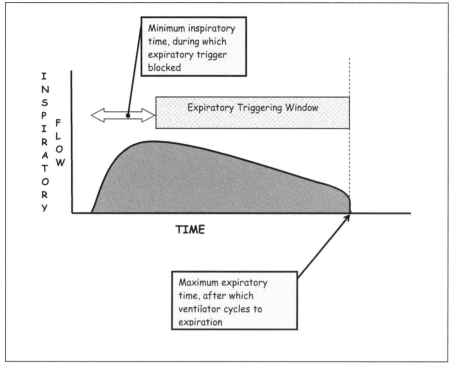

Figure 26.4 The expiratory trigger window.

Most of the time, you won't need to touch the triggers on an NIV ventilator. When you are using pressure-control you don't really want the patient to be triggering many breaths themselves — the whole idea is for the ventilator to do most of the work. With bi-level pressure-support for acute respiratory failure, most patients will be fine with standard trigger settings.

Mask leaks and triggering

Mask leaks have a bad effect on triggering. If the patient starts to take a breath in, most of the air comes from around the mask and is not sensed by the ventilator, which therefore fails to trigger inspiration. If the flow rate during inspiration is very high because of leaks, the reduction in the flow into the patient as their lungs fill up is only a small proportion of the excessively high flow. The ventilator is looking for a proportional fall in flow, say to 70% of maximum. This will not happen, with air just pouring out of the leaks, so inspiration will be terminated by time-cycling rather than flow-cycling.

Key Point	Terminology	**Practical Tip**	Physiology	How to do it

Before you start adjusting trigger sensitivity, make sure that the mask fit is as good as you can get it.

Key Point	Terminology	Practical Tip	Physiology	**How to do it**

Adjust triggers
- Check the mask and minimise leaks first before you adjust the triggers
- Watch the patient on NIV
- If they are having to make quite an effort to trigger a breath in, make the inspiratory trigger more sensitive
- Watch again, and check that the setting is not so sensitive that the ventilator is sensing a breath when there isn't one (autotriggering)
- The expiratory trigger needs to be more sensitive if the patient is having to contract their expiratory muscles to turn off inspiration, or if there is a long pause after the lungs are fully inflated before the switch to expiration occurs
- To make the expiratory trigger more sensitive, increase the flow level at which the switch to expiration occurs
- Watch again, and check that inspiration is not now too short

Summary

- Most modern ventilators use flow to trigger the start of inspiration
- During bi-level pressure-support, expiration is triggered when inspiratory flow falls below a certain level
- Mask leaks interfere with these triggers

27
Oxygen

Learning points

By the end of this chapter you should be able to:

- Explain how you decide when to use supplementary oxygen with NIV
- Describe where the oxygen port should be inserted in an NIV circuit

NIV is mainly used to correct hypoventilation. Provided the lungs themselves are in reasonable shape, oxygenation should improve as $PaCO_2$ comes down. There will also be less shunting through atelectatic areas of lung, for example in the lower lobes of patients with diaphragm weakness, since IPAP will increase ventilation to these regions.

If you start NIV without supplemental oxygen, you can use SpO_2 as an indicator of whether you have established effective alveolar ventilation.

Key Point	Terminology	**Practical Tip**	Physiology	How to do it

Start NIV without supplemental oxygen and see what happens to the SpO_2. If it remains below 90%, try increasing the IPAP before you reach for the oxygen.

Target SpO$_2$

If there is no reason to suspect lung disease, aim for an SpO$_2$ of 94-98%. In someone with chronic hypercapnia, 88-92% is a better target. You might think that it doesn't matter about abolishing respiratory drive by giving too much oxygen to someone who is on NIV, but in practice they will be having breaks from NIV for meals etc., when they will be breathing by themselves.

The other situation when you may opt for the lower of these two ranges is in the presence of lung or pulmonary vascular disease, when there is little chance of you getting the SpO$_2$ above 88-92%. You may even choose a lower range still, say 80-85%, in severe lung disease such as COPD. Remember that it is unaccustomed hypoxia that causes problems.

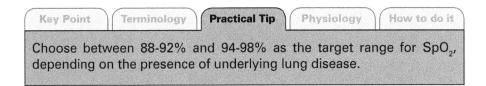

| Key Point | Terminology | **Practical Tip** | Physiology | How to do it |

Choose between 88-92% and 94-98% as the target range for SpO$_2$, depending on the presence of underlying lung disease.

Oxygen blenders

Critical care ventilators are usually connected to piped oxygen, with a blender in the ventilator which gives a precise FiO$_2$. The oxygen concentration remains constant no matter how high the flow rate delivered by the ventilator.

This is particularly important in two situations:

- **When you need to regulate FiO$_2$ carefully, for example in a patient with COPD**
- **When you need a high FiO$_2$, for example in a patient with lung disease and type 1 respiratory failure**

Supplementary oxygen ports

For most other NIV ventilators, you will need to put a connector into the circuit and connect this with some tubing to your oxygen source. Inserting the connector at the ventilator end of the circuit is neater. You don't then have oxygen tubing around the bed, hanging off the patient end of the circuit and getting tangled up. Oxygen accumulates in the circuit, so that when the patient takes a breath in, they inhale this reservoir of oxygen-enriched air.

Alternatively, attach the oxygen tubing directly to the mask. When you are using bi-level NIV, if you insert an oxygen connector to the patient end of the circuit there is a risk that most of the oxygen gets blown out of the expiratory port. Make sure it is between the patient and the expiratory port, or put it at the ventilator end of the circuit

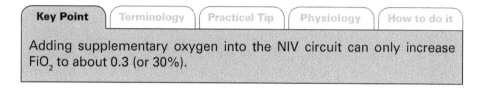

Key Point	Terminology	Practical Tip	Physiology	How to do it
Adding supplementary oxygen into the NIV circuit can only increase FiO_2 to about 0.3 (or 30%).				

Humidification

Oxygen is always a dry gas, whether it comes from a piped supply, concentrator or cylinder. If you are using oxygen with a humidifier, it makes sense to add it to the inspired gas at a point where it will pick up moisture from any humidification device you are using.

EPAP and oxygenation

EPAP is good for oxygenation, in that it should prevent basal atelectasis and hence improve ventilation-perfusion matching. When you add EPAP, the mean pressure in the airways is increased, and this provides a driving pressure to help "push" oxygen across from the alveoli into the blood. The down side is that adding EPAP reduces ventilation, so you need to be sure that you still have enough alveolar ventilation to keep $PaCO_2$ down. EPAP will also blow supplementary oxygen out of the expiratory port, hence reducing FiO_2.

Overnight oxygenation

There is no real need to check overnight oxygen saturation if, after starting NIV, your patient is sleeping well, daytime PaO_2 is >8 kPa and $PaCO_2$ has improved. However, it's easy to do and many centres check it routinely in patients on long-term NIV. If you don't, there are a couple of things that should make you think of checking the oxygen saturation overnight. The first is right heart failure and the second is polycythaemia. In both these conditions it is good to get the mean SpO_2 above 90% if you can.

NIV and LTOT in COPD

As we discussed in Chapter 13, sometimes the only way you can establish a patient with COPD onto LTOT without pushing the $PaCO_2$ dangerously high is to use NIV.

| Key Point | Terminology | Practical Tip | **Physiology** | How to do it |

Causes of hypoxia

- Hypoventilation: If you don't get any air into your lungs, you go blue. We get a bit fixated with hypoventilation leading to hypercapnia, and sometimes forget that it is an important cause of hypoxia also

- Ventilation-perfusion (V/Q) mismatch: This is the most important cause of hypoxaemia. As an extreme case, if all the blood were going to one lung and all the air to the other then there would be no gas exchange. Lesser degrees of V/Q mismatch are the explanation for most of the hypoxia we see in clinical practice

- Impaired diffusion: In healthy lungs, diffusion of oxygen across the alveolar-capillary membrane is completed within about 0.25 seconds. This is fast enough, since the red blood cells are in the pulmonary capillaries for about 0.75 seconds. If there is a block to diffusion, for example in fibrosis, diffusion may take much longer. As a result, red cells leave the pulmonary capillaries before they have become fully saturated (Figure 27.1)

- Shunt: Blood that passes from the right side of the heart to the left, for example through an atrial or ventricular septal defect, will not be oxygenated in the lungs. The same thing happens with intra-pulmonary arterio-venous malformations.

cont ...

Key Point | Terminology | Practical Tip | **Physiology** | How to do it

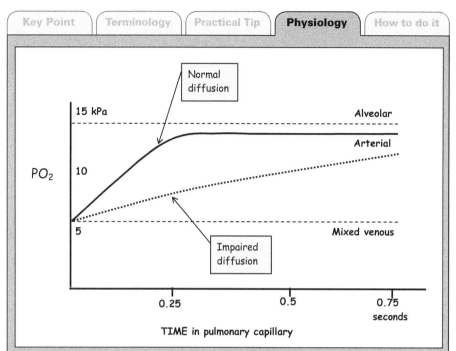

Figure 27.1 Diffusion block as a cause of hypoxaemia. Normal diffusion gets the blood oxygen levels up to arterial in 0.25s. If diffusion is impaired, this may not have happened by the time the blood leaves the pulmonary capillaries (about 0.75s). Exercise shortens the time spent in the capillaries to about 0.25s. This exacerbates hypoxaemia if diffusion is impaired.

Even in normal lungs, there is some degree of V/Q mismatch. Similarly, everyone has a small shunt. We could add these to our oxygen cascade from Figure 2.6 (Figure 27.2).

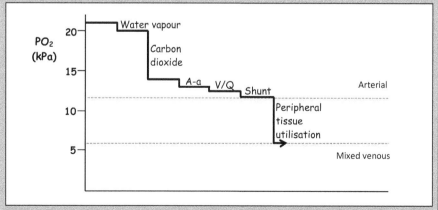

Figure 27.2 The oxygen cascade, from inspired air to arterial blood.

Summary

- **For acute respiratory failure, the best way of adding oxygen in NIV is to use a ventilator with an oxygen blender**
- **For home NIV, entrain oxygen through a port in the circuit**

28
Obesity-Hypoventilation Syndrome

Learning points

By the end of this chapter you should be able to:

- **Describe how to select patients with obesity-hypoventilation syndrome for long-term NIV**
- **Set up NIV for these patients**
- **Explain about respiratory drive**

During REM sleep, ventilation is provided by the diaphragm. In an obese subject asleep in the supine position, the weight of abdominal fat pushing up into the chest may cause hypoventilation. When you measure lung volumes in obesity, a low functional residual capacity (FRC) is the commonest finding. We've already seen that this results in low oxygen stores to buffer apnoeas (chapter 23).

The commonest respiratory problem related to obesity is obstructive sleep apnoea (OSA), causing sleep deprivation from recurrent arousals and mild daytime hypercapnia, which will resolve with CPAP.

| Key Point | **Terminology** | Practical Tip | Physiology | How to do it |

Obstructive sleep apnoea
During an obstructive apnoea, there is continued respiratory effort but no airflow because the upper airway is occluded. The obstructive sleep apnoea syndrome additionally requires the presence of symptoms, most importantly daytime sleepiness.

Some obese patients (about 10%) who do not have OSA nevertheless slip into hypercapnic respiratory failure. They have poor respiratory drive. This will be even worse during sleep. Combined with the mechanical effects of obesity on respiration, they will first develop hypercapnia during sleep, whilst maintaining normal daytime $PaCO_2$. Eventually they become hypercapnic during the day as well. This is termed obesity-hypoventilation syndrome (OHS).

| Key Point | Terminology | **Practical Tip** | Physiology | How to do it |

An obese patient with a normal daytime $PaCO_2$ but elevated bicarbonate is likely to have nocturnal hypoventilation.

OSA or OHS?

How do you decide whether a sleepy obese individual, with a history of snoring and apnoeas, has OSA alone or OHS with OSA? If the daytime $PaCO_2$ is very high, say greater than 8 kPa, it is likely to be OHS. Overnight oximetry may show a low baseline, on which obstructive episodes are superimposed. Transcutaneous CO_2 monitoring will tell you if there is hypercapnia. More detailed studies including airflow and thoraco-abdominal motion will help you sort out if there is a central component to any apnoeas. Better still, just watch the patient when they are asleep.

| Key Point | Terminology | **Practical Tip** | Physiology | How to do it |

If you're not sure if a patient has OSA or OHS, start them on NIV rather than CPAP. If it turns out to be mainly OSA, you can step them down to CPAP at a later stage.

COPD and OHS

Many of the patients with COPD who do well on NIV are pretty overweight. They are "blue bloaters" rather than "pink puffers". Actually, they sometimes turn out to have COPD that isn't all that bad, and the cause of hypoventilation was more one of central respiratory drive. The term "overlap syndrome" is sometimes used for OHS and COPD in the same patient. I prefer to list both separately, with the emphasis on OHS as the main cause of their hypercapnia.

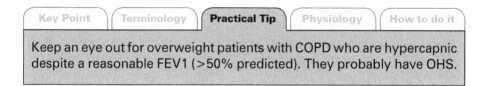

| Key Point | Terminology | **Practical Tip** | Physiology | How to do it |

Keep an eye out for overweight patients with COPD who are hypercapnic despite a reasonable FEV1 (>50% predicted). They probably have OHS.

Which patients?

Patients with OHS usually present with acute or acute-on-chronic type 2 respiratory failure. Daytime $PaCO_2$ will be high, with a bicarbonate >30 mmol/l. In these patients, just as in those with scoliosis or neuromuscular problems, it doesn't matter what the pH level is: they need NIV. (Daytime hypercapnia is unlikely if their VC is >3 litres and SpO_2 >94%).

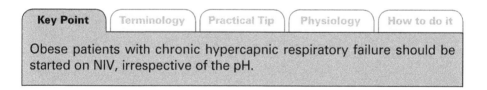

| **Key Point** | Terminology | Practical Tip | Physiology | How to do it |

Obese patients with chronic hypercapnic respiratory failure should be started on NIV, irrespective of the pH.

The safest policy is to start NIV straight away. Don't be fooled by how well they look — if you do nothing then you are highly likely to get a call from ICU a few days later. Similarly, it is worth considering nocturnal NIV in an obese patient who has transient hypercapnic respiratory failure during an acute illness. If it has only taken a minor respiratory tract infection to tip them over, this is highly likely to happen again soon. Most of them will be back within a year.

Obese patients with an elevated $PaCO_2$ are likely to need NIV at night in the long term.

Ventilator settings

Start with bi-level pressure-control, but be prepared to switch to IPPV if the patient doesn't pick up quickly. Respiratory drive is poor in these patients, particularly at night, so they will be using the back-up settings most of the time. Pressure-support ventilators are designed to support rather than provide ventilation, and they don't do the latter as well. If the patient takes very short shallow breaths at a rate above the back-up rate, the ventilator supports these breaths, but they may not provide adequate alveolar ventilation.

We've noted that it can be difficult to decide if a patient has OSA, OHS or a mixture of both. Obviously OSA requires CPAP, whilst IPPV may be better for pure OHS. Bi-level pressure-control or support fit somewhere in the middle (Figure 28.1).

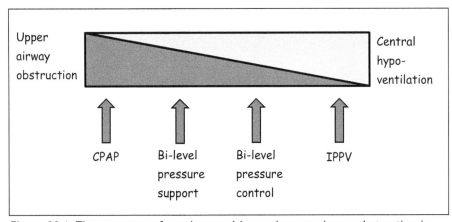

Figure 28.1. The spectrum of respiratory drive and upper airway obstruction in obesity.

Patients with OHS are at risk of underventilation if you put them on pressure-support, because of their poor respiratory drive.

Start with an IPAP of 15 cmH$_2$O or so, but push it up fairly soon to 20 cmH$_2$O once the patient is settled. If they will tolerate it, you can use even higher IPAP, up to about 30 cmH$_2$O. An EPAP of 5 cmH$_2$O is fine to start with, but if the patient is very obese and oxygenation or upper airway obstruction is a problem, then you can increase it. Bear in mind that if you push the EPAP up a lot, NIV starts to look more like high pressure CPAP (Figure 28.2, compared to Figure 2.2).

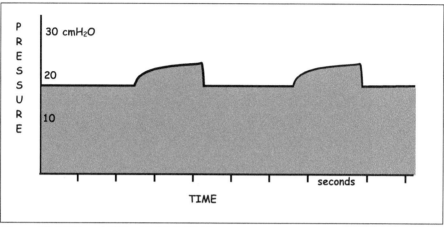

Figure 28.2 Bi-level NIV with high EPAP.

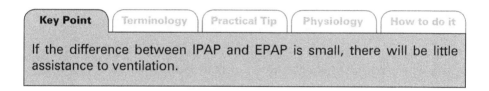

Key Point | Terminology | Practical Tip | Physiology | How to do it

If the difference between IPAP and EPAP is small, there will be little assistance to ventilation.

Set a reasonably high back-up rate (12 to 15 breaths/min) with an I:E ratio of 1:2 (unless the patient also has COPD, when 1:3 would be better).

Where?

These patients have often experienced a slow decline into respiratory failure, and tolerate terrible arterial blood gases surprisingly well. They are often fine on a respiratory ward, but the very sick ones should be on HDU.

How long for?

Very occasionally, a patient with obesity-hypoventilation will lose a massive amount of weight and be able to stop using NIV. Most patients will need to continue with nocturnal NIV indefinitely.

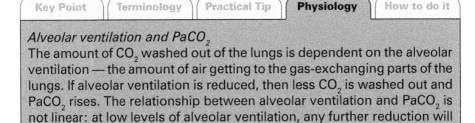

| Key Point | Terminology | **Practical Tip** | Physiology | How to do it |

It is extremely rare for patients with OHS to lose enough weight to be able to stop using NIV.

| Key Point | Terminology | Practical Tip | **Physiology** | How to do it |

Alveolar ventilation and PaCO$_2$
The amount of CO$_2$ washed out of the lungs is dependent on the alveolar ventilation — the amount of air getting to the gas-exchanging parts of the lungs. If alveolar ventilation is reduced, then less CO$_2$ is washed out and PaCO$_2$ rises. The relationship between alveolar ventilation and PaCO$_2$ is not linear: at low levels of alveolar ventilation, any further reduction will result in a much larger rise in PaCO$_2$ (Figure 28.3).

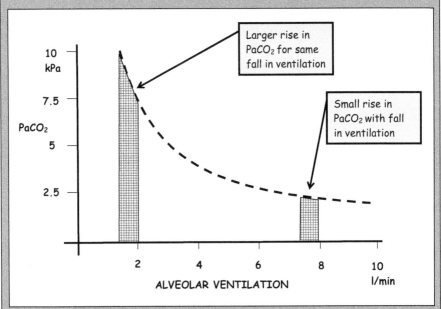

Figure 28.3 A similar change in alveolar ventilation will result in a much larger change in PaCO$_2$ if alveolar ventilation is already low.

Summary

- Obesity-hypoventilation is likely to become the commonest reason for using long-term NIV at home
- If the patient needs NIV acutely, they probably need it long-term
- Use IPPV or pressure-control

29
Palliative Care

Learning points

By the end of this chapter you should be able to:

* **Explain which end-of-life symptoms can be helped by NIV**
* **Outline how you would withdraw NIV**

Sometimes we may suggest a trial of NIV towards the end of life, with a specific therapeutic goal in mind. Sometimes for a patient who has been on NIV for some time, we gradually switch the emphasis from an active to a palliative approach. In both contexts it is important to be clear about what you are trying to achieve with NIV (Figure 29.1).

Hypercapnia is universal at the end of life. Since we tell everyone that the best treatment for hypercapnia is NIV, it is perhaps not surprising that we get asked so often to start it when this would clearly be inappropriate. The patient's symptoms may not be amenable to NIV, or they may not even have any. Knowing what NIV can and cannot do will help you in these situations.

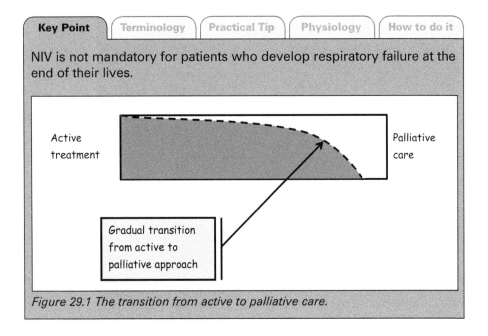

| Key Point | Terminology | Practical Tip | Physiology | How to do it |

NIV is not mandatory for patients who develop respiratory failure at the end of their lives.

Active treatment

Palliative care

Gradual transition from active to palliative approach

Figure 29.1 The transition from active to palliative care.

Breathlessness

NIV can be a good way of relieving breathlessness, for example in a patient with MND and tired inspiratory muscles. Bear in mind that if it works well there is a real risk that the patient will become dependent on the ventilator, with the problem then of how to come off NIV.

Always consider other ways of relieving breathlessness before resorting to NIV, for example draining a pleural effusion. It may also be more appropriate to use other non-drug measures, or medication such as opiates or benzodiazepines. NIV can be very intrusive towards the end of life, particularly in preventing communication. Ask yourself if there is a realistic chance that NIV will work, then ask the patient if they want to try it. Explain to them the implications for them of becoming ventilator-dependent. Use this opportunity to discuss an end-of-life care plan.

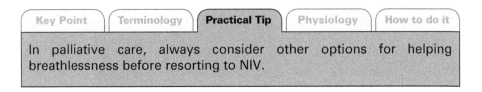

| Key Point | Terminology | Practical Tip | Physiology | How to do it |

In palliative care, always consider other options for helping breathlessness before resorting to NIV.

You may not have the opportunity to have these discussions. Some patients with severe COPD start NIV for an acute exacerbation, but then find as the days go by that they can't come off it even for a few minutes. It is the only thing that helps their breathlessness. This usually means they have very severe disease and have come to the end of their life.

Sleep disturbance

Severe respiratory muscle weakness is often associated with poor sleep, as we have already discussed. NIV is particularly helpful in maintaining adequate ventilation at night and allowing restorative sleep. (Some patients with respiratory muscle weakness may use NIV for this indication for months or years.) If sleep disturbance is a prominent symptom towards the end of life, and you feel that there is a realistic chance it is the result of hypoventilation, it may be worth doing a sleep study (or offering a therapeutic trial of NIV).

Therapeutic trials

Once the goal of care is clear, try NIV. Some patients will like it. Others won't. If the treatment is worse than the original symptoms, then just stop NIV. It's up to the patient to decide. Don't press on with NIV when they clearly hate it.

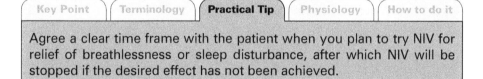

| Key Point | Terminology | **Practical Tip** | Physiology | How to do it |

Agree a clear time frame with the patient when you plan to try NIV for relief of breathlessness or sleep disturbance, after which NIV will be stopped if the desired effect has not been achieved.

Prolongation of life

NIV has the potential to prolong life. This is mainly relevant to patients with neuromuscular disease, who can live for months or years longer because of NIV. In COPD patients with their final exacerbation, NIV can keep them alive for a few more days. Rather than the patient saying, "I want to live longer, so I'll start NIV", it is much more common for them to find themselves on NIV and be thinking, "If I stop this, I won't live as long as if I stay on it". Either way, it is up to the patient to decide if they want to live longer. If they don't, we can plan with them how to withdraw NIV. If they don't have capacity, or have not made an advance decision to refuse treatment, we must act in their best interests.

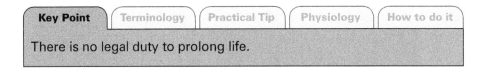

Key Point Terminology Practical Tip Physiology How to do it

There is no legal duty to prolong life.

Futility

Futility is a key concept in palliative care. It is futile to continue NIV if it is not achieving what it is intended to do. We may have a physiological goal, for example improvement in $PaCO_2$. If this is not achieved, we may decide that NIV is futile. The patient's goal will be different, such as relief of breathlessness or better sleep. If NIV doesn't improve the symptom, it's futile. If you stop NIV, explain to the patient that you will move on to explore other options to help them. This is a bit like switching medication to find something that works. It doesn't mean you are giving up on them.

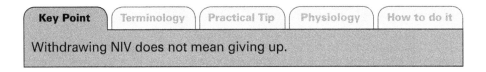

Key Point Terminology Practical Tip Physiology How to do it

Withdrawing NIV does not mean giving up.

Withdrawal of NIV

There is often a lot of anxiety about withdrawing NIV. You may need to spend quite a bit of time with the team, making sure that everyone understands the ethical and legal issues. It can help to point out to colleagues that when someone dies, it is the underlying illness that is the cause of death, not the fact that you stopped NIV — a healthy subject would not die if you had them on NIV then stopped it.

Anticipatory prescribing

Patients and their families or carers often worry that withdrawing NIV may lead to distressing symptoms. It often doesn't. Nevertheless, make sure appropriate medication is prescribed. If distress or breathlessness is likely, administer appropriate medication (anxiolytic, perhaps with an opiate for breathlessness) before you stop NIV. Explanation, reassurance and compassion are just as important as drugs.

There is sometimes confusion about the "double effect" of drugs such as opiates, where relief of a distressing symptom is associated with respiratory depression which may expedite death. The intention is solely to relieve the symptom. The need to do so is sufficient reason to produce the bad effect. Studies of the use of drugs at the end of life suggest that the negative impact of opiates and benzodiazepines is generally overestimated.

Advance decisions to refuse treatment

It is becoming increasingly common for patients to have a legally-binding document which states their wishes in terms of medical treatment. This can include instructions about withholding or withdrawing NIV. Such documents are invaluable when the patient has deteriorated to a stage where they lack the capacity to make such decisions themselves. If they do have capacity, then they can let you know at the time if their wishes have changed — it is perfectly reasonable for them to change their minds.

| **Key Point** | Terminology | Practical Tip | Physiology | How to do it |

Advance decisions to refuse treatment (ADRTs) are only of relevance when the patient no longer has the capacity to make decisions about their treatment.

| Key Point | Terminology | Practical Tip | Physiology | **How to do it** |

Assess capacity to refuse NIV
- Start with the presumption that the patient has capacity, until proven otherwise
- In assessing capacity, do not be influenced by the patient's appearance, age, mental health diagnosis, disability or medical diagnosis
- Be prepared to allow the patient to make what you might feel is an unwise decision, if they have the capacity to do so
- Define the clinical decision that is being made
- Explain the options and implications of that decision to the patient
- Check that they understand what you have told them
- See if they have retained the information for long enough to make a decision
- Ask them what they want to do
- If they are unable to easily communicate their decision to you, explore other ways for them to do so
- Document each stage of this process in the patient's records

If the patient states that they do not wish to have NIV, or have a valid ADRT in place stating that they do not wish to be treated with NIV, then in law it would be classified as assault to start NIV.

| Key Point | Terminology | **Practical Tip** | Physiology | How to do it |

Withholding and withdrawing a treatment have the same legal status, but on the ground they feel very different.

| Key Point | Terminology | Practical Tip | Physiology | **How to do it** |

Withdraw NIV
- Explain to the patient, family, carers and staff what you plan to do and why. Address any concerns before you proceed
- If you think it is highly likely that the patient will experience distressing symptoms when you stop NIV, administer medication (an anxiolytic and an opiate) and wait for an appropriate interval
- Sit with the patient
- Silence the ventilator alarms
- When they are ready, take off the NIV mask
- Start them on supplementary oxygen straight away. You can stop this within a few minutes if it proves to be unnecessary
- Stay with the patient
- If they become distressed, put them back on NIV and try again in a few minutes. Consider further doses of medication
- Once the patient is settled off NIV, turn the ventilator off. Leave it by the bedside until you (and the patient) are sure that they aren't going to need it
- If they can't manage even a few breaths off NIV, change from pressure-control to pressure-support and reduce the IPAP to the lowest level that relieves symptoms
- Some patients may want to hold the NIV mask for themselves, putting it on and off at their own pace

Best interests

In a patient who lacks capacity, make a decision that is in their best interests. Take into account any previously-expressed wishes of the patient. Talk to the carers, family; anyone who might have anything to contribute to the decision.

You might think that "best interest" decisions are about withdrawing NIV. But every time you start NIV on an acutely ill patient who is too ill to participate in decision-making, you are acting in their best interests. If you do act on the basis of best interest, this should be the least restrictive option available to you. You will have little hesitation in starting NIV in a drowsy patient for whom it is clearly the right thing to do. If they are delirious and start pulling the mask off, you would have to consider more "restrictive" options. If you are thinking of using sedation, or even physical restraint, then at the very least get a second opinion. An independent mental capacity advocate may be helpful in this situation.

Key Point	Terminology	Practical Tip	Physiology	How to do it

When acting in the patient's best interests, rather than with their explicit consent, you must use whichever option is open to you that has the least restrictive effect on their liberty.

Decision regret

Decisions made in uncertainty are prone to decision regret. For the patient this is fine, because they can change their mind at any time. You must remind them that they can. Relatives, however, may be left with feelings of guilt. At the risk of sounding paternalistic, I think it is up to us as professionals to take responsibility for these decisions. We should seek the support of the relatives, but do not burden them with making the decisions.

Summary

- NIV can be very effective in relieving symptoms at the end of life
- Don't use it if the patient doesn't want it
- Withdrawing NIV is morally and legally acceptable

30
Humidification

Learning points

By the end of this chapter you should be able to:

- Explain the factors that limit how much water vapour air can contain
- Differentiate between a bacterial filter and a heat-moisture exchanger
- Draw the circuit for using a heated water-bath humidifier with NIV
- Draw the circuit for using a heated-wire humidifier with an NIV ventilator

Most of the time humidification isn't necessary with NIV. The nose is designed to humidify inspired air, and does this pretty well for patients using a nasal mask or nasal pillows. With an oro-nasal mask, there may be some dryness of the mouth which is a bit of a nuisance. Occasionally it may be the factor which limits the use of NIV. In this situation you may wish to try humidification.

Heat and moisture exchangers

One of the simplest ways of increasing the amount of moisture in the inspired gas is to trap the water vapour (and heat) from the exhaled air in a device that is a bit like a sponge, then pass the air from the ventilator through this before it goes to the patient. This is called a heat and moisture exchanger (HME). Since the sponge also traps bacteria, it is often called an HME filter (Figure 30.1).

Key Point	**Terminology**	Practical Tip	Physiology	How to do it

An HME filter is a wad of material that traps heat and moisture from the expired air, then adds it to the inspired air.

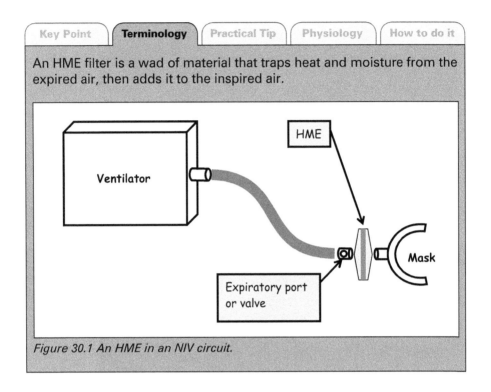

Figure 30.1 An HME in an NIV circuit.

Key Point	Terminology	**Practical Tip**	Physiology	How to do it

Make sure that the HME is positioned in the circuit so that expired air passes through it.

One problem with an HME is that the material may become saturated with water. The wad of damp material in the filter then greatly increases resistance to flow. This may affect triggering, since it is more difficult for the ventilator to detect the small increase in flow which tells it that the patient wants to start a breath.

When a ventilator blows air along the circuit, it expects to experience resistance from the patient's lungs. The resistance to flow is what forces the ventilator to produce a pressure — remember how we had to produce a pressure to inflate our balloon right at the start of this book? If there were no balloon then you could blow out with very little pressure. An HME may provide enough resistance to produce a significant pressure in the circuit. The ventilator senses this, and can be fooled into thinking it has produced enough pressure to inflate the patient's lungs. To see this effect, put an HME filter on the end of a ventilator without attaching it to a patient and look at the ventilator display to see what sort of pressures are being generated.

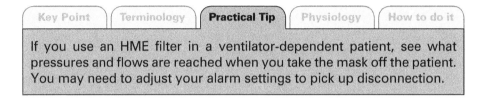

Key Point | Terminology | **Practical Tip** | Physiology | How to do it

If you use an HME filter in a ventilator-dependent patient, see what pressures and flows are reached when you take the mask off the patient. You may need to adjust your alarm settings to pick up disconnection.

Heated humidifier

The amount of water air can contain is dependent on temperature. Warm air can hold more moisture, which is why condensation forms when you breathe out onto a window pane — the air cools down when it hits the window, and can no longer hold as much moisture, so water droplets form.

Some patients can only tolerate NIV if they have a bit more moisture. Passing the inspired air over a heated water chamber will usually do the trick. This just requires an extra section of 22 mm tubing (Figure 30.2).

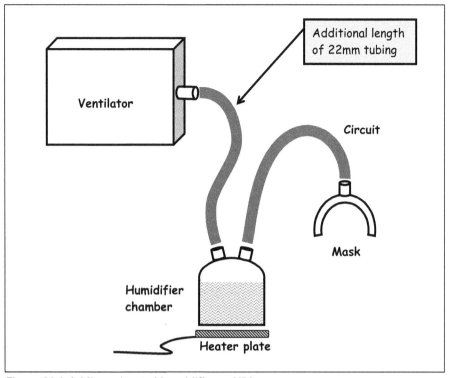

Figure 30.2 Adding a heated humidifier to NIV.

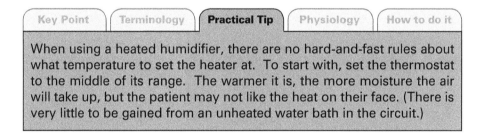

| Key Point | Terminology | **Practical Tip** | Physiology | How to do it |

When using a heated humidifier, there are no hard-and-fast rules about what temperature to set the heater at. To start with, set the thermostat to the middle of its range. The warmer it is, the more moisture the air will take up, but the patient may not like the heat on their face. (There is very little to be gained from an unheated water bath in the circuit.)

Heated wire humidifiers

Not many patients with NIV need humidification with a heated wire circuit, but let's take a quick look at them anyway whilst we're on the subject. You are more likely to come across this sort of humidification when a "non-invasive" ventilator is used with a tracheostomy.

A heated humidifier chamber gets moisture into the air from the ventilator, but as the air flows down the circuit towards the patient the temperature falls. Water condenses and accumulates in the circuit. This is called "rain out". To minimise this, we can put a wire down the inside of the circuit and heat it up to keep the air warm. We'll need a temperature gauge at the end of the circuit where it goes into the mask, to make sure we don't make the air too hot (34°C is a reasonable target). All this adds to the complexity of the circuit, with the possibility of disconnection, leaks or failure of triggering (Figure 30.3).

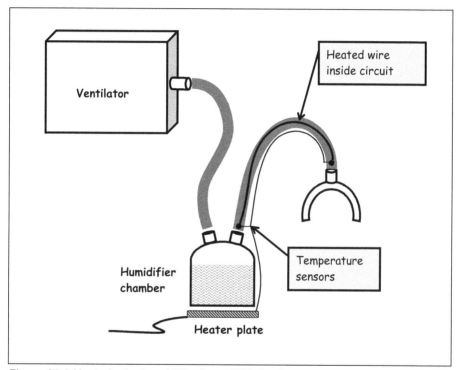

Figure 30.3 Heated wire humidifier in an NIV circuit.

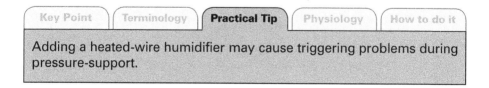

Adding a heated-wire humidifier may cause triggering problems during pressure-support.

Summary

- Humidification isn't usually necessary with NIV, since the upper airway will humidify the inspired air
- Heat-moisture exchangers (HMEs) can affect how the ventilator works
- Some patients will only tolerate NIV if they have a heated water chamber to humidify the inspired air
- Heated-wire humidifiers are seldom needed with NIV

31
Ventilator– Patient Synchronisation

Learning points

By the end of this chapter you should be able to:

* **Spot when a patient is not synchronising with NIV**
* **Work out how to rectify the situation**

It is quite common to be asked to see a patient with acute respiratory failure on NIV and find that the ventilator and the patient are completely out of time with each other. The team looking after them will look at the ventilator display and the arterial blood gases but fail to notice that the patient is not receiving effective ventilatory support. If they are getting better, it is despite having the ventilator blowing IPAP at them when they are breathing out. Take them off NIV and they'll probably just continue to improve. If they are not getting better, we need to work out the reason for failure of synchronisation and do something about it.

Key Point	Terminology	Practical Tip	Physiology	How to do it

The first thing to do when looking at a patient on NIV is to watch carefully to check that the ventilator is synchronising with their own spontaneous respiratory efforts.

Mask fit

Suppose the NIV mask was lying on the bed, there would be no way the ventilator would be able to detect when the patient started to breathe in. Put the mask loosely on their face, with loads of leaks, and the ventilator will still struggle to sense the change in flow that indicates the start of inspiration. Good triggering relies first and foremost on a good mask fit with minimal leaks.

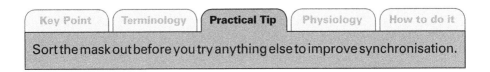

Key Point	Terminology	**Practical Tip**	Physiology	How to do it

Sort the mask out before you try anything else to improve synchronisation.

Failure of inspiratory triggering

When we use NIV in a patient with acute respiratory failure, our aim is for the ventilator to deliver IPAP in time with the patient's own inspiratory effort. For the onset of each breath the ventilator must detect the start of inspiratory flow, and then rapidly introduce IPAP in order to take over the work of breathing. You can check this by watching the patient's neck muscles. As soon as you see any activity in the muscles, the ventilator should kick in straight away.

When you look at the patient, it is easily apparent if the patient is completely out of time with the ventilator. If not, look more carefully to see if the patient is having to work quite hard to trigger the ventilator. Is there a short delay? It may only be a tenth of a second, but this is uncomfortable for the patient and they will be wasting a lot of inspiratory muscle effort.

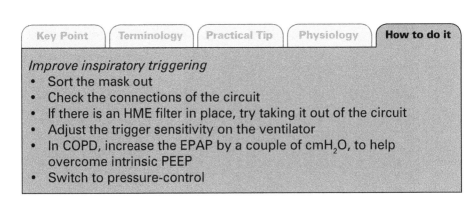

Key Point	Terminology	Practical Tip	Physiology	**How to do it**

Improve inspiratory triggering
- Sort the mask out
- Check the connections of the circuit
- If there is an HME filter in place, try taking it out of the circuit
- Adjust the trigger sensitivity on the ventilator
- In COPD, increase the EPAP by a couple of cmH_2O, to help overcome intrinsic PEEP
- Switch to pressure-control

Autotriggering

Ventilators sometimes get confused. If the patient has taken off their mask and put it down on the bed, the ventilator may be racing along much faster than the back-up rate you would expect it to run at. This is called autotriggering, with the ventilator sensing a breath when there isn't one. It is all to do with the high flow rate down the tubing, causing swings in pressure and flow which the ventilator misinterprets.

When the ventilator is attached to a patient, autotriggering is unusual. Look out for it if you have increased the sensitivity of the inspiratory trigger. Check what the back-up rate of the ventilator is set at and watch to see if it is putting in any extra breaths, not clearly triggered by the patient.

Failure of expiratory triggering

When the patient is ready to breathe out, the ventilator must sense this and rapidly switch over to expiration. If the ventilator continues to blow IPAP when the patient is clearly trying to breathe out, consider making the expiratory trigger more sensitive. Check the fit of the mask first. Some ventilator modes allow you to set a minimum inspiratory time during pressure-support, which in this case may be too long.

Sleep

What happens when our patient drops off to sleep? Their mouth falls open or their head slumps forward and the mask starts to leak. We're back to square one. The ventilator struggles to sense when the patient wants to breathe and we get completely out of time. Many ventilators will now allow you to download data to show how much asynchrony there is overnight.

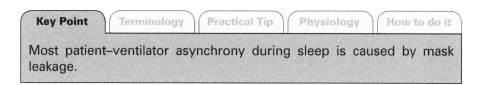

Key Point	Terminology	Practical Tip	Physiology	How to do it

Most patient–ventilator asynchrony during sleep is caused by mask leakage.

Try and sort the mask out, but often this is impossible to fix completely. Adjust the trigger sensitivity. A different approach has been advocated whereby triggering is done using electrodes to detect electrical activity in the respiratory muscles — electromyography (EMG). This is attractive because it happens very early on in inspiration and doesn't require the ventilator to detect flow. However, EMG signals are tiny voltages that are very prone to interference, so it's not really a viable option in clinical practice.

Upper airway obstruction

Closure of the upper airway obviously prevents the ventilator from sensing when the inspiratory muscles are trying to start the next breath. If you watch a patient on NIV when they are asleep, maybe someone with obesity-hypoventilation, there will be times when the chest doesn't move. They then have the sort of arousal from sleep that you will probably have seen on sleep studies. They open up their pharynx, after which the chest moves up and down nicely in time with when the ventilator applies IPAP. If you see this happen, re-positioning the patient's head may be all that is necessary. Switching to bi-level ventilation and pushing up the EPAP may also work. In severe OSA, it is sometimes necessary to use an EPAP of 15 or even 20 cmH$_2$O.

Pressure-control

When we use NIV longer term, we want the ventilator to do all the work, with the patient resting their respiratory muscles. So we don't them to have to trigger each breath, and we certainly don't want them to be fitting breaths in completely out of time with the ventilator.

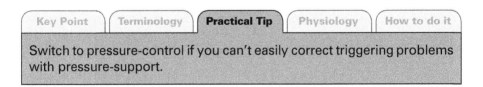

| Key Point | Terminology | **Practical Tip** | Physiology | How to do it |

Switch to pressure-control if you can't easily correct triggering problems with pressure-support.

Summary

- With pressure-support, de-synchronisation between the ventilator and the patient is quite common
- Mask leak is often the cause

32
Inspiratory: Expiratory Ratio

Learning points

By the end of this chapter you should be able to:

- Set the I:E ratio for back-up breaths in pressure-support according to the presence or absence of airflow obstruction
- Set the I:E ratio for pressure-control
- Explain how short expiratory times lead to hyperinflation
- Calculate the I:E ratio from respiratory rate and inspiratory time

During tidal breathing, you spend about a third of the time breathing in, then a third breathing out; the final third is a pause before the next breath in. If one third of the breathing cycle is spent breathing in and two thirds breathing out (including the pause as part of expiration), this gives an I:E ratio of 1:2.

When a patient develops breathing problems, they pinch time from the pause between breaths and start the next breath as soon as the previous breath finishes. If they have a problem with getting air out of the lungs, for example COPD, the pause will be used for expiration. If the problem is getting air into the lungs, for example in neuromuscular weakness, more time will be spent in inspiration.

During spontaneous breathing, patients automatically breathe with the I:E ratio which is most efficient for them. With pressure-support, the ventilator will allow them to breathe with this pattern too, except for back-up breaths. Use a ratio of 1:2 for the back-up breaths, or 1:3 if the patient has airflow obstruction.

Key Point	Terminology	Practical Tip	Physiology	How to do it

With pressure-support, the I:E ratio setting only applies to back-up breaths.

Pressure-control

• **Inspiratory time**

Start with the same time as the patient takes for a spontaneous breath. Watch the patient carefully on NIV (and/or look at the volume-time trace on the ventilator if there is one) and adjust the inspiratory time so that it is just long enough for the lungs to reach full inflation. If you try and prolong inspiration too much, then the patient will start to feel uncomfortable and start to fight the ventilator. Once the patient is settled, you will probably be able to slow the rate down. One way of doing this is just to increase the inspiratory time a little. If you watch the patient, you will probably be able to see that the chest expands better. There comes a point, however, where the chest has expanded as much as it is going to for that IPAP — prolonging inspiration further will be uncomfortable for the patient, even though it might allow time for air to get into the bits of lung with long time constants (see Physiology).

Alveolar time constants

Stiff areas of lung — with reduced compliance — have short time constants and are sometimes called "fast" alveolar units. They inflate very quickly. A high elastic recoil pressure (which is the same thing as reduced compliance) stops airways collapsing, so this part of the lung will also empty very quickly.

With a rapid respiratory rate, more ventilation will go to these "fast" parts of the lung. They may not be very good at getting oxygen across into the blood compared to the "slower" areas of normal lung (Figure 32.1).

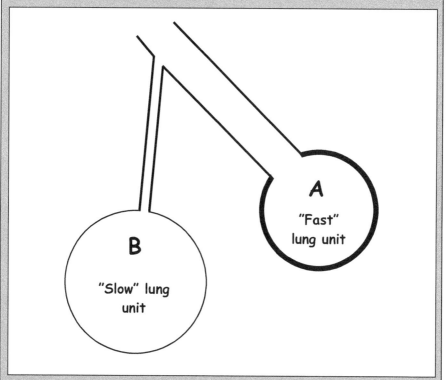

Figure 32.1. The time taken to inflate alveoli with low compliance is shorter than for normal areas of lung.

Just to complete the picture, in COPD there will be very slow alveolar units, with long time constants. This is because they have narrow airways and very compliant (emphysematous) alveoli.

- **Expiratory time**

Someone with fairly normal lungs will have completed expiration in about a second or two. In severe COPD, expiration may take three seconds or more. It is essential that you leave enough time for these patients to exhale, but again this should be apparent by watching the patient carefully. If you have the luxury of a flow trace, you can see whether or not expiratory flow falls to zero before the next breath in (Figure 32.2).

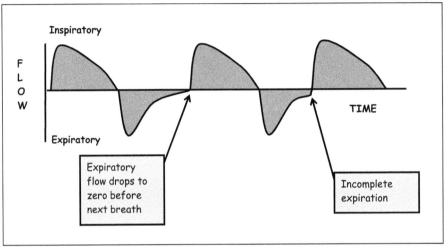

Figure 32.2 Expiratory flow. Inspecting the expiratory flow on the flow-time trace will show you if there is sufficient time for expiration to finish before the next breath. This applies for "control" breaths — during pressure-support the patient will determine the optimal expiratory time for themselves.

If you don't allow the patient to complete expiration, you will progressively hyperinflate them. PEEPi will become more of a problem (see "Triggering"). Try breathing for a minute or so just below total lung capacity rather than your normal lung volume — it is uncomfortable, and harder work for your inspiratory muscles.

Short expiratory time and re-breathing

Just for completeness, it is worth remembering that with bi-level NIV the exhaled air is blown out through the expiratory port during expiration. If the expiratory time is too short, there is a theoretical risk of re-breathing exhaled air that has not been flushed out of the circuit.

Key Point	**Terminology**	Practical Tip	Physiology	How to do it

I:E ratio
Some ventilators give you the respiratory rate, then allow you to adjust the I:E ratio. For example, if you choose a rate of 15 breaths per minute, each breath will be four seconds long; an I:E ratio of 1:3 means inspiration would last one second and expiration three seconds. Other ventilators get you to set the inspiratory and expiratory times separately. So we might set inspiration to 1.5 seconds and expiration to 3 seconds; total breath time is 4.5 seconds, the I:E ratio is 1:2 and the rate is just over 13 breaths per minute (60/4.5).

Summary

- I:E ratio means the ratio of the time spent in inspiration to that spent in expiration
- Don't worry too much about I:E ratios on pressure-support — they only apply to the back-up rate
- In pressure-control, set the I:E ratio to the pattern of spontaneous breathing for that patient
- In COPD you will need a long expiratory time, and you may need to shorten the inspiratory time to get an appropriate I:E ratio

33
Type 1 Respiratory Failure

Learning points

By the end of this chapter you should be able to:

- Identify patients with type 1 respiratory failure who might benefit from NIV
- Ensure that NIV for these patients is delivered in an appropriate clinical area
- Describe how you would bronchoscope a patient on NIV

NIV helps with ventilation rather than oxygenation, but some patients with type 1 respiratory failure (low PaO_2, normal or low $PaCO_2$) seem to benefit. The evidence suggests that it is better to start it early, and then intubate if NIV fails. NIV doesn't work at all well when it is used as a last-ditch option, when the patient has been turned down for intubation by ICU, on a "nothing to lose" basis.

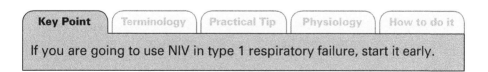

Key Point	Terminology	Practical Tip	Physiology	How to do it

If you are going to use NIV in type 1 respiratory failure, start it early.

Which patients?

The list of conditions involving type 1 respiratory failure for which NIV has been documented to be effective is getting longer and includes pneumonia, trauma, adult respiratory distress syndrome (ARDS), severe acute respiratory syndrome (SARS) and asthma. The level of evidence for the use of NIV in these conditions is not yet particularly high, although there is an accumulating body of evidence in immunocompromised patients with diffuse lung infiltrates.

Key Point	Terminology	Practical Tip	**Physiology**	How to do it

PF ratio (PaO_2/FiO_2 ratio)
A slightly low PaO_2, say 10 kPa (normal range 10-13 kPa), may not seem too bad if your patient is breathing room air (with 21% oxygen, or an FiO_2 of 0.21). If they are on 100% oxygen (FiO_2 1.0) then the implication is that they have a much more serious problem. We could work out the A-a gradients (see later section in this chapter), but a quicker way to see how well they are absorbing oxygen is to calculate the PF ratio. The P is PaO_2, the F is FiO_2. A PaO_2 of 10 kPa on 100% oxygen gives a PF ratio of 10/1.0. The same PaO_2 on room air gives a PF ratio of around 50 (10/0.2). You can see that the lower the PF ratio, the worse the problem with oxygenation. A PF ratio lower than 40 is used to define acute lung injury, lower than 25 is ARDS.

Key Point	Terminology	**Practical Tip**	Physiology	How to do it

A low PF ratio is one of the things which predict failure of NIV in type 1 respiratory failure, particularly if it fails to improve quickly once you start NIV. The worse the problem with oxygenation, the less likely NIV is to work.

Some of the other adverse predictors will sound familiar from our discussions about COPD:

- pH <7.2
- Pneumonia on CXR
- Severe physiological disturbance
- Inability to get PF ratio above 25
- Low BMI
- Low GCS

Key Point | Terminology | Practical Tip | Physiology | **How to do it**

Bronchoscope during NIV
You may need to bronchoscope a patient whilst they are on NIV, either to lavage in order to get a diagnosis in a patient with diffuse infiltrates, or to remove a plug of sputum which is causing a segment of lung to collapse.

- Obtain consent
- Keep the patient nil-by-mouth for four hours before the procedure
- Decide if it is going to be safe to use sedation
- Make sure you have good intravenous access
- Check all the endoscopic equipment carefully before you start
- Make sure everything you might possibly need is at hand
- Turn the supplementary oxygen up to maximum
- Insert a bronchoscopy connector (available from ICU) where the circuit attaches to the mask. If you have one available, use a special NIV bronchoscopy mask or helmet
- Double-check that everything is ready
- Insert the bronchoscope
- Be as quick as you can. If you have prepared carefully, you can do a bronchoalveolar lavage in a minute or so. Getting plugs of sputum out of a collapsed lobe may take longer

Ventilator settings

Use bi-level pressure-support. Since the patient has difficulty with oxygenation, you will need to use a high EPAP such as 10 cmH$_2$O. The lungs are stiff, so IPAP may need to be a bit higher to increase ventilation, say 25 cmH$_2$O.

Supplementary oxygen

In type 1 respiratory failure, you will need supplementary oxygen. Ideally you want an SpO$_2$ of 94-98%. Adding oxygen into the circuit can only get FiO$_2$ up to about 0.3 (30%). A ventilator with an oxygen blender is a much better option in this situation to deliver a precise FiO$_2$.

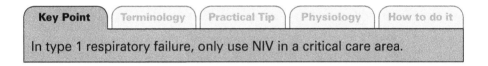

Key Point | Terminology | Practical Tip | Physiology | How to do it

In type 1 respiratory failure, use an NIV ventilator which has its own oxygen blender.

Where?

There is a high likelihood of needing to intubate, so patients with type 1 respiratory failure should receive NIV on ICU. If intubation is not an option, it may be appropriate to use HDU. These patients may become severely hypoxic if their mask comes off, so they should not be managed on a lower intensity facility such as a general or respiratory ward.

Key Point | Terminology | Practical Tip | Physiology | How to do it

In type 1 respiratory failure, only use NIV in a critical care area.

How long for?

As with COPD, it should be apparent within a few hours whether NIV is going to work. If gas exchange has not improved after four hours, you should probably stop.

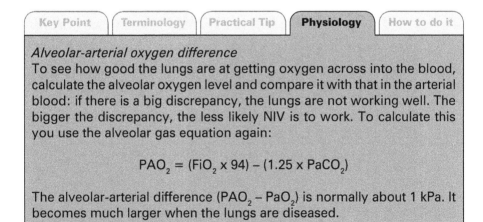

Key Point | Terminology | Practical Tip | **Physiology** | How to do it

Alveolar-arterial oxygen difference
To see how good the lungs are at getting oxygen across into the blood, calculate the alveolar oxygen level and compare it with that in the arterial blood: if there is a big discrepancy, the lungs are not working well. The bigger the discrepancy, the less likely NIV is to work. To calculate this you use the alveolar gas equation again:

$$PAO_2 = (FiO_2 \times 94) - (1.25 \times PaCO_2)$$

The alveolar-arterial difference ($PAO_2 - PaO_2$) is normally about 1 kPa. It becomes much larger when the lungs are diseased.

cont...

Key Point | Terminology | Practical Tip | **Physiology** | How to do it

The most important cause of an elevated A-a gradient is ventilation/perfusion imbalance. The reason for this is simple to understand if you look at the two alveolar units in Figure 33.1, one of which is very poorly perfused (Unit A) and the other of which is poorly ventilated (Unit B). Since there is very little perfusion of Unit A, the composition of gas within it will be quite similar to inspired air — the PAO_2 will be high, and the (limited volume of) blood leaving the unit will be well oxygenated. On the other hand, Unit B is underventilated, so the blood leaving the unit is little different from the blood entering it — poorly-oxygenated mixed venous blood. So, we have well-oxygenated blood leaving Unit A and poorly-oxygenated blood leaving Unit B. The two sources of blood mix together in pulmonary veins, ready to be transported round the arterial system. We already noted that Unit A was under-perfused, so most of the blood comes from Unit B which is poorly oxygenated.

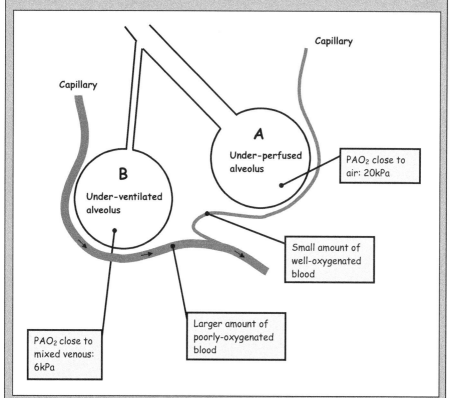

Figure 33.1 Ventilation/perfusion imbalance. A larger proportion of the blood entering the systemic arterial system comes from Unit B which is underventilated but well-perfused, in comparison with Unit A which is well-ventilated but under-perfused.

Summary

- The lower the PF ratio, or the higher the A-a gradient, the less chance there is of NIV working
- IPAP and EPAP will need to be quite high, e.g. 25/10 cmH$_2$O
- In type 1 respiratory failure, use a ventilator with an oxygen blender
- Manage patients on ICU or HDU

34
Complications

Learning points

By the end of this chapter you should be able to:

- List potential complications of NIV
- Add a humidifier to an NIV circuit
- Plan how you would assess and reduce the risk of complications in your unit

Serious complications of NIV are pretty rare. Skin problems and nasal symptoms are more common, and often limit how much NIV your patient will tolerate.

Nasal bridge pressure sores

The most common complication is skin ulceration because of pressure from the mask. The bridge of the nose has very little tissue between the cartilage and the skin, and can easily become red or ulcerated within a few hours on NIV particularly if the mask straps are very tight. Prevention is better than cure. Don't over-tighten masks. If the skin starts to become red, change to a different style of mask before ulceration develops — this might be a smaller mask which fits over the tip of the nose, one with a pad which sits on the forehead to relieve pressure on the nasal bridge, or some nasal pillows. Some units routinely apply a small square of protective dressing such as Granuflex® to the bridge of the nose in a patient starting NIV acutely who is likely to have a mask on for most of the first 24 hours.

Nasal symptoms

Sneezing is sometimes a problem when a patient first starts NIV, probably because the higher flow rates during ventilation cool down the nose. Some patients on long-term NIV continue to experience lots of nasal symptoms, such as stuffiness or a runny nose. Steroid or anticholinergic nasal sprays may be helpful. They should be tried for several weeks, applied to each nostril twice daily. Other simple measures include an insulating sleeve around the ventilator tubing, or putting a few drops of decongestant in the bacterial filter each night. If none of these measures work, increasing the humidity of the inspired air may be worth a try. You could use an HME or heated humidifier (see Chapter 30).

Sinus pain

Some patients experience pain in their sinuses during NIV. Apart from reducing the IPAP, it is difficult to do much about this. Heated humidifiers may help.

Irritation of eyes

If a mask fits badly, sometimes the air blowing into the eyes can cause irritation. Try a better-fitting mask, or a different sort of interface.

Gastric distension

When you apply pressure to the upper airway through a mask, most of the air will go into the lungs but some may go down into the oesophagus. Most patients on long-term NIV learn to stop this from happening, although quite how they do so is not clear. It may help to reduce the IPAP. For some patients, this problem never seems to go away.

Oesophageal/gastric perforation

There have been occasional reports of oesophageal rupture on NIV, in patients who had a spontaneous perforation some years previously. Traditionally, it was thought that NIV should not be used soon after oesophageal or gastric surgery. It has now been established that NIV after gastric surgery for obesity is safe.

Pneumothorax

Pneumothorax as a complication of NIV is extremely rare, but is something to bear in mind if a patient deteriorates suddenly. It is more likely to occur in someone with bullous or cystic lung disease. It is possible to continue with NIV in the presence of a small pneumothorax, but it is much safer to insert a chest drain.

Facial shape

Use of a mask for hours at a time will distort the shape of the face, particularly in children. Nasal pillows may cause dilation of the anterior nares. Prolonged use of a mouthpiece can alter the alignment of teeth. Rotating through several types of interface is the only way of preventing these problems in patients who are highly dependent on NIV.

Summary

- Serious complications of NIV are rare
- Nasal bridge pressure is the most common problem

35
Failure of NIV

Learning points

By the end of this chapter you should be able to:

* **Decide what to do when your patient is not improving on NIV**
* **Explain when and how you would use sedation with NIV**

After an hour or so, a patient you have started on NIV should begin to improve. Often this is apparent from the end of the bed, in that they no longer look as if they are fighting to stay alive. An arterial blood gas sample will tell you if your clinical impression is right. If the pH level and $PaCO_2$ are moving in the right direction, then you need do nothing more — changing the ventilator settings or mask may well unsettle the patient, just when they are getting used to NIV.

Sometimes the patient seems to be better when you look at them and their gases are also improving, but when you watch them being ventilated it is clear that NIV is not working. They may be out of synchronisation with the ventilator, or there may be lots of leaks and the target pressure isn't being achieved, or they are just unhappy about the whole thing and are trying to pull the mask off the whole time. In this case they are improving despite rather than because of NIV, and you should discontinue it.

What if the patient does not look any better and their arterial blood gases are not improving? It may be best to abandon NIV, but there are a few things to check first.

Key Point	Terminology	Practical Tip	Physiology	How to do it

There is always a danger of persevering with NIV too long. Don't delay intubation if it is apparent that NIV is not going to work.

Is the patient synchronising with the ventilator?

If the patient is not synchronising with the ventilator, then NIV will not be achieving anything, and may even be making the situation worse. The most common problem is mask leak, but there are a few other things you could try:

- Check the circuit is connected correctly. If you are using an exhalation valve, check that the smaller tubes are connected at both ends, and not blocked by water or secretions
- Check that the filter has not become clogged with water or secretions
- Increase the inspiratory trigger sensitivity
- Increase EPAP if the patient has COPD, to overcome PEEPi
- If the patient is breathing very fast, shorten the rise time
- Increase the EPAP if you think there is upper airway obstruction. This is more likely to occur when the patient is asleep. See what happens if you change the position of the patient's head, if you pull their jaw forward or if you wake them up. You may need to sit them more upright. A nasopharyngeal airway may help if the patient's conscious level is impaired

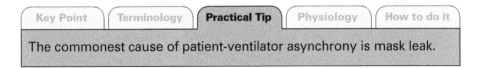

Key Point	Terminology	**Practical Tip**	Physiology	How to do it

The commonest cause of patient-ventilator asynchrony is mask leak.

Is the chest expansion adequate?

If the chest is expanding in time with the ventilator but the $PaCO_2$ is not improving:

- Think about re-breathing: check the patency of the expiratory port; use a different port
- Increase the IPAP
- Decrease the EPAP. This will increase span and hence Vt
- With pressure-control, increase the inspiratory time
- With pressure-control (or if the back-up rate is being used on pressure-support) increase the respiratory rate
- Change ventilator mode. If you are not winning on pressure-support, try pressure-control. If these pressure-targeted modes aren't working, some patients will pick up on volume ventilation, but set a clear time limit on further trials of different modes

Is medical therapy optimal?

Check that you have ordered all the appropriate medication, and that it has been given. It is easy to overlook things that you would routinely give if the patient wasn't on NIV. If it has been difficult to settle the patient onto NIV, there may not have been time to give them all their drugs. If the oxygen flow rate is too high, you may lose the patient's own contribution to ventilation. Aim for an SpO_2 of 88-92%.

Have any complications developed?

Although very unlikely, it is always worth thinking about the possibility of a pneumothorax. If in doubt, get a chest X-ray. New lung shadowing might also indicate that the patient has aspirated.

Would sedation help?

Very occasionally you may need to try sedating the patient to see if this improves their tolerance of NIV, but only do this if you are not going to proceed to intubation, or if you are in an environment where the patient can be intubated rapidly if things deteriorate.

| Key Point | Terminology | Practical Tip | Physiology | **How to do it** |

Sedate a patient on NIV
- Use the intravenous route
- Give small incremental doses every few minutes
- Use a drug whose effect you can completely reverse, such as a benzodiazepine
- Make sure the reversing agent is by the bedside
- Remember that the half-life of the reversing agent is much shorter than the sedating drug — you may need to use repeat doses or even an infusion

Withdrawing NIV and palliative care

If the patient's clinical condition and their blood gases are deteriorating despite optimal NIV and a decision has been made not to intubate, then you should stop NIV. Do this as soon as it is clear that NIV is failing. The longer you delay this decision the more difficult it will be to stop NIV. The patient will usually be relieved to take off the mask. Sometimes they feel very breathless without NIV, but it is better to use oxygen, opiates or benzodiazepines to manage this rather than go back onto NIV. If the patient is dying, it is important that they are able to talk to their family and to the staff caring for them — NIV makes this difficult. It may also draw out the process of dying and prolong suffering.

It can be difficult to know how quickly a patient will deteriorate when you stop NIV, so make sure that all the right people are around.

If the patient cannot cope with stopping NIV so suddenly, try reducing the IPAP slowly. If you can get it down to less than 10 cmH$_2$O, the switch to spontaneous breathing may be less abrupt. This sounds kinder, but the whole process runs the risk of becoming very drawn out. NIV can prolong as well as alleviate suffering.

Summary

- If a patient is not improving on NIV, watch them closely for a few minutes and diagnose the problem
- If corrective action doesn't work, consider changing ventilator mode
- The decision to intubate or palliate will depend on whether effective ventilation has been established with NIV

36
Cervical Cord Lesions

Learning points

By the end of this chapter you should be able to:

- Explain how the level of a cervical cord lesion affects the likelihood of developing respiratory failure
- Describe the indications for NIV in spinal cord injury

High cervical cord transection

I'm sure you will know that the diaphragm is innervated from cervical nerve roots C3, 4 and 5. Complete transection of the spinal cord above C3 leaves only a few neck muscles for respiration, so full-time ventilator support will be necessary. This usually means invasive ventilation via a tracheostomy.

Low cervical cord transection

If the transection is at C6 or lower, diaphragm function is preserved and the patient is usually able to maintain adequate ventilation. Occasionally these patients need NIV. Look out for symptoms of hypoventilation during sleep, recurrent episodes of hypercapnic respiratory failure, or even just recurrent chest infections. It is not unusual for these patients to have symptoms for several years before someone gets round to offering them a trial of NIV. This is particularly likely when the spinal level is not clear.

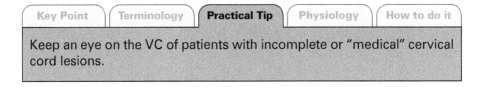

| Key Point | Terminology | **Practical Tip** | Physiology | How to do it |

Many patients have incomplete lesions, involving mid-cervical segments in a patchy way. They will have some spontaneous ventilation, but it is easy to miss them slipping into ventilatory failure. Check their daytime bicarbonate level and do a sleep study.

Progressive lesions

When cervical cord transection is the result of trauma, it may take a few months for the spinal level to settle to its final point. With "medical" cord lesions (syringomyelia, inflammation or a tumour), remember that the neurology may progress. Ask about new symptoms and re-examine regularly. VC is the best test to tell you if respiratory muscle involvement is getting worse.

| Key Point | Terminology | **Practical Tip** | Physiology | How to do it |

Keep an eye on the VC of patients with incomplete or "medical" cervical cord lesions.

Non-invasive ventilation

Use bi-level pressure-control. (The EPAP will prevent basal atelectasis). Unless the patient is obese, 15-20 cmH$_2$O will be enough IPAP. For respiratory rate and I:E ratio, start with something similar to the patient's own spontaneous pattern. Once they are settled, slow down the rate a bit and prolong inspiratory time slightly. Nasal masks are the best first option for nocturnal use. Think about mouthpieces for daytime NIV top-ups.

Key Point \ Terminology \ Practical Tip \ **Physiology** \ How to do it

Ribcage paradox

In order to breathe in, we need a negative pressure inside the thoracic cage. Normally, the external intercostals and diaphragm both contribute to the generation of the necessary negative pressure. The intercostals expand the ribcage by producing the "bucket handle" upwards and outwards motion of the ribs.

If the inspiration is purely generated by the diaphragm, as is the case with low cervical cord transection, the only force acting on the ribcage is the negative pressure inside the chest. As a result, during inspiration it moves inwards, rather than upwards and outwards. This is called paradoxical ribcage motion (Figure 36.1).

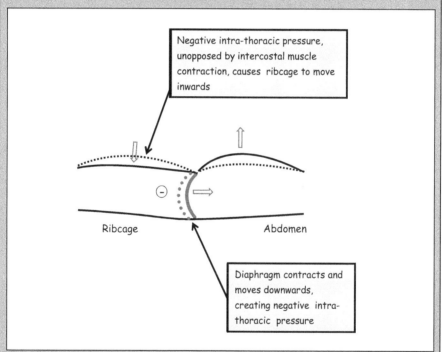

Negative intra-thoracic pressure, unopposed by intercostal muscle contraction, causes ribcage to move inwards

Ribcage   Abdomen

Diaphragm contracts and moves downwards, creating negative intra-thoracic pressure

Figure 36.1 Paradoxical inward motion of the ribcage when the diaphragm generates a negative intra-thoracic pressure.

You can feel this for yourself if you put a hand on your sternum and suck in hard against a closed glottis. This is because the diaphragm is stronger than the intercostals. A similar mechanism explains the change in phase of ribcage and abdominal motion during obstructive sleep apnoea.

Summary

- **NIV is a good treatment for patients with lower cervical cord lesions who develop lots of chest infections**
- **Use pressure-control**

37
Leaks

Learning points

By the end of this chapter you should be able to:

- **Describe how leaks affect NIV**
- **Explain some measures that can be used to minimise leaks**

We've talked quite a lot about leaks. They are one of the main issues we face with NIV. Let's go back over some of the problems they cause.

Comfort

Mask leaks are uncomfortable. They make a noise, which can be a problem for the patient or their bed-partner. The leaking air feels cold. It can cause corneal irritation.

IPAP

NIV ventilators are designed to cope with leaks, but they have their limits. If the leak is too great, the target IPAP will not be reached.

Triggering inspiration

In pressure-support modes, the ventilator needs to detect a change in flow in order to decide when to start a triggered breath. When the patient starts to take a breath, some of the inspiratory flow occurs through the leaks around the mask. It is more difficult for the ventilator to pick up inspiratory effort.

Triggering expiration

Ventilators cycle to expiration when they detect a fall in the rate of flow of air into the lungs, implying that the lungs are nearly full. This is more difficult to detect if the overall flow rate is very high because of leaks.

Oxygen

A critical care ventilator will have an oxygen blender, so the air it delivers to the patient will always have the correct proportion of oxygen. If you are using a simpler ventilator with an oxygen port in the circuit, leaks force the ventilator to blow more air, whereas the oxygen flow remains the same. As a result, the inspired oxygen concentration falls.

Humidification

A humidifier has a limited capacity to get water into the inspired gas. If the flow rate is high, the humidity will be less.

Estimation of Vt

Many NIV ventilators will provide an estimate of Vt. They do this by guessing that, for any given pressure, there will be a certain amount of leakage. The higher the pressure the greater the leak. But the leak isn't measured, so this is really a guesstimate. The greater the leak, the less accurate this estimate is likely to be.

Summary

- **Leaks are a problem**
- **They are uncomfortable**
- **They interfere with the function of the ventilator**

38
Muscle Diseases

Learning points

By the end of this chapter you should be able to:

- **List some examples of neuromuscular diseases which lead to chronic type 2 respiratory failure**
- **Decide when a patient with one of these diseases needs NIV**

We talked earlier on about splitting patients who need NIV into two main groups:

1. Patients with common diseases who present with acute hypercapnic respiratory failure and need NIV for a few hours or days during the acute illness (mainly COPD).
2. Patients with fairly normal lungs who slip into hypercapnic respiratory failure because their breathing muscles give up or their central respiratory drive is poor (ventilatory pump failure).

Numerically, patients with ventilatory pump failure are much less common than our first group, but they are important to think about because a high proportion will need NIV subsequently at home. Long-term survival in these patients is often excellent, for example over 80% at five years in scoliosis or stable neuromuscular conditions, so it is important that you know how to get them through the initial crisis.

Just to re-cap, type 2 respiratory failure — failure of ventilation — can occur because the load on the respiratory muscles is too great, because the muscles are weak with a reduced capacity to perform work, or because the respiratory drive to maintain a normal $PaCO_2$ is not working properly. In this chapter, we're mainly concerned with the second of these three situations — reduced muscle capacity (Figure 38.1).

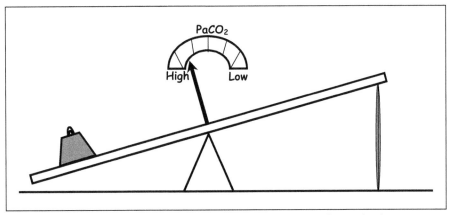

Figure 38.1. The balance between load and capacity determines whether a normal PaCO$_2$ can be maintained.

There are many diseases which can affect the respiratory muscles, either because the muscles themselves are involved, or because there is a problem with the nerves or neuromuscular junction. The end result is the same — respiratory muscles which don't contract. The clinical picture will depend upon which respiratory muscles are not working, and the degree of weakness.

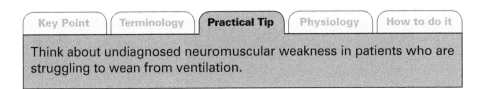

Key Point | Terminology | **Practical Tip** | Physiology | How to do it

Think about undiagnosed neuromuscular weakness in patients who are struggling to wean from ventilation.

Vital capacity

The simplest way to assess respiratory muscle weakness is to measure VC. It is a robust test, using readily available equipment. If you see a patient with a muscle disease, measure VC. If it is greater than 3.0 litres, respiratory failure is very unlikely at that point in their illness. If they have a disease which is not likely to affect their respiratory muscles, you can probably just ask them to come back and see you if they develop respiratory symptoms.

If their disease is on your list of patients to watch (see below), arrange to measure VC again in a year. When it falls to 1.5 litres, see them every six months.

Once VC is down to 0.75 litres or less, respiratory muscle weakness is becoming critical. Reduce the interval to 3 months and keep a much closer eye out for signs and symptoms of hypoventilation. Have a low threshold for doing an arterial blood gas and/or a sleep study.

Key Point	Terminology	**Practical Tip**	Physiology	How to do it

If the vital capacity (VC) of a patient with a neuromuscular problem is greater than 3.0 litres, the risk of them developing ventilatory failure is low.

Respiratory muscle strength

As a general rule, hypercapnic respiratory failure is unlikely in this group of patients unless inspiratory muscle strength is less than 50% predicted. This corresponds to a maximal inspiratory pressure (MIP) or sniff nasal inspiratory pressure (SNIP) of about 40 cmH_2O (4 kPa).

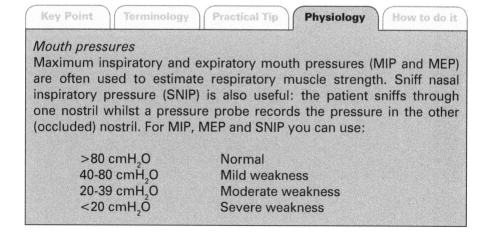

Key Point	Terminology	Practical Tip	**Physiology**	How to do it

Mouth pressures
Maximum inspiratory and expiratory mouth pressures (MIP and MEP) are often used to estimate respiratory muscle strength. Sniff nasal inspiratory pressure (SNIP) is also useful: the patient sniffs through one nostril whilst a pressure probe records the pressure in the other (occluded) nostril. For MIP, MEP and SNIP you can use:

>80 cmH_2O	Normal
40-80 cmH_2O	Mild weakness
20-39 cmH_2O	Moderate weakness
<20 cmH_2O	Severe weakness

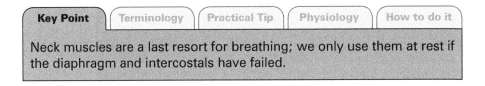

| Key Point | Terminology | **Practical Tip** | Physiology | How to do it |

Keep a close eye on those patients with muscle diseases who have a VC <0.75 litres or an MIP <20 cmH$_2$O.

Watching the patient breathe can be more informative than doing tests. Look and see if the patient is using their accessory muscles (sternomastoid etc.) to breathe at rest — a sign that all the main respiratory muscles are very weak — and count the respiratory rate: 30 breaths or more per minute implies that the muscles are so weak that Vt is small and the only way the patient can get a reasonable minute ventilation is by breathing very fast.

| **Key Point** | Terminology | Practical Tip | Physiology | How to do it |

Neck muscles are a last resort for breathing; we only use them at rest if the diaphragm and intercostals have failed.

From time to time you will come across patients who use rocking to breathe spontaneously. All their respiratory muscles have gone, but by using their paraspinal and abdominal muscles they can rock to and fro. This uses the abdomen as a piston to pump a small amount of air in and out of the lungs. Clearly this is a sign of severe respiratory muscle weakness — time for nocturnal NIV, if they are not on it already.

Hypercapnia

We try very hard to keep our PaCO$_2$ within the normal range, so if a patient with neuromuscular disease is hypercapnic during the daytime it means they have very weak respiratory muscles and will need NIV as a matter of urgency.

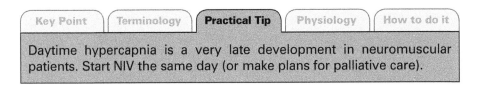

| Key Point | Terminology | **Practical Tip** | Physiology | How to do it |

Daytime hypercapnia is a very late development in neuromuscular patients. Start NIV the same day (or make plans for palliative care).

We all underventilate slightly when we are asleep; in neuromuscular disease, significant hypercapnia is often first present during sleep, and only manifests during the daytime as the disease progresses. Nocturnal awakenings and excessive daytime sleepiness may alert you to nocturnal hypoventilation in a patient, but the symptoms can be very vague — fatigue, poor appetite, weight loss, poor concentration, personality change.

Muscle diseases

NIV works well in patients with muscle disorders such as muscular dystrophy. The classification of these disorders is evolving with the discovery of new genetic defects. Those which are particularly prone to affect the respiratory muscles are:

- **Duchenne muscular dystrophy**
- **Acid maltase deficiency**
- **Limb-girdle muscular dystrophy**
- **Nemaline myopathy**

You are likely to think about respiratory muscle weakness when the patient is already in a wheelchair because of limb muscle problems, but remember that some muscle diseases may have respiratory failure as their presenting problem. Some examples of muscle diseases where respiratory failure may occur when the patient is still ambulant are:

- **Acid maltase deficiency**
- **Emery-Dreifuss myopathy**
- **Nemaline myopathy**
- **Mitochondrial myopathy**
- **Limb-girdle muscular dystrophy (type 2i)**
- **Minicore myopathy**

It isn't necessary (or possible, for most of us) to remember all the details of these different diseases, but you need to keep a closer eye on patients with a condition on any of the above two lists. An annual VC will be fine initially. When the VC falls below 1.5 litres, consider seeing them more often. An annual sleep study is also advisable at this stage. We used to wait until the patient had symptoms attributable to nocturnal hypoventilation before doing sleep studies, on the grounds that "prophylactic" NIV in patients without sleep disturbance was seldom tolerated. The problem is that these symptoms are sometimes very vague, and they creep up on patients without them realising. Also, we now know that patients with neuromuscular diseases with asymptomatic nocturnal hypoventilation will be in trouble within a year or so. It is much better to start NIV before there is a crisis.

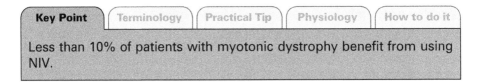

| Key Point | Terminology | **Practical Tip** | Physiology | How to do it |

Remember to do regular echocardiograms on patients with muscle conditions that may affect the heart: Duchenne, Becker, Emery-Dreifuss and limb-girdle (type 1b) muscular dystrophies.

Myotonic dystrophy

This is the commonest muscle disease. Daytime sleepiness is almost invariable, usually as part of the disease process rather than disruption of sleep by underventilation. If you do overnight oximetry on a sleepy myotonic dystrophy patient you will see periods of desaturation related to REM sleep. Starting NIV doesn't tend to make them feel any better. If you look at compliance with NIV in myotonic dystrophy, less than 10% use it for 4 hours or more in the longer term.

| **Key Point** | Terminology | Practical Tip | Physiology | How to do it |

Less than 10% of patients with myotonic dystrophy benefit from using NIV.

There are, however, a small number of patients with myotonic dystrophy who develop hypercapnic respiratory failure which responds well to NIV, which is subsequently used to good effect long term. Spotting these patients who do well on NIV is quite difficult when they first present. It's much easier when you look at the compliance data on the ventilator one month later.

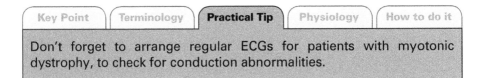

| Key Point | Terminology | **Practical Tip** | Physiology | How to do it |

Don't forget to arrange regular ECGs for patients with myotonic dystrophy, to check for conduction abnormalities.

Neuralgic amyotrophy

One disease which you will come across from time to time is neuralgic amyotrophy. This is an inflammatory condition affecting the brachial plexus. After a non-specific prodromal phase, the patient develops pain in the shoulder and breathlessness. Clinical examination may reveal wasting of shoulder muscles on the side of the pain, with paradoxical abdominal motion indicating bilateral diaphragm paralysis. It is not clear if both phrenic nerves become inflamed at the same time, or whether one side has been affected previously without much in the way of symptoms, breathlessness only occurring when the other side goes. (It is not uncommon to see an asymptomatic elevated hemi-diaphragm on a CXR). Spontaneous recovery is slow and unpredictable. Orthopnoea and sleep disturbance are common symptoms in this condition. They respond well to NIV.

Ventilator settings

IPPV is usually the best mode of NIV to use in neuromuscular patients. (Use bi-level pressure-control if you haven't got the option of IPPV.) Even the effort of triggering the ventilator on and off is a considerable burden for these patients, and it is better to take over breathing for them completely. Set the respiratory rate slightly lower than their own rate, and think about adjusting this down as they improve. Patients with neuromuscular diseases are often very relieved to get onto NIV, and spontaneous respiratory effort will cease if you get their settings right. The chest will be fairly easy to inflate, so an IPAP of 18 cmH$_2$O may be sufficient.

Bi-level pressure-support is designed to support breathing rather than provide ventilation, and the back-up settings are only there as a safety measure. Neuromuscular patients will generate shallow, short breaths, particularly during sleep when the pattern may also be very irregular; the ventilator will support these breaths, but ventilation may well be inadequate because of the short inspiratory time unless spontaneous breathing stops altogether and the back-up settings kick in.

EPAP makes triggering easy for COPD patients, but we aren't asking our neuromuscular patients to trigger the ventilator. EPAP will help keep the lungs inflated and overcome basal atelectasis, but pressure-controlled ventilation will also be adequate for this. For very weak patients, the effort of overcoming even a low EPAP can be quite a struggle.

| Key Point | Terminology | **Practical Tip** | Physiology | How to do it |

Patients with neuromuscular problems have pretty compliant chests, so be careful not to overventilate them.

Summary

- Patients with muscle diseases are at risk of hypoventilation once their VC is <0.75 litres
- If they have daytime hypercapnia they need NIV urgently
- Use pressure-control modes with a modest IPAP

39
Acute Neurological Syndromes

Learning points

By the end of this chapter you should be able to:

- Give an example of an acute neurological illness in which NIV may be needed
- Describe how you would set up NIV for them
- Explain when invasive ventilation would be more appropriate

There are some neurological diseases which cause acute paralysis which then improves either spontaneously or with treatment — polymyositis, ascending neuropathy (Guillain-Barré syndrome), myasthenia etc. If ventilatory failure develops, intubation or tracheostomy is usually necessary. This is safer than NIV, with protection of the airway against aspiration. As respiratory muscle function becomes progressively worse, there will be a stage when NIV may just be enough to maintain adequate ventilation safely, but most patients rapidly progress through this stage. If you do decide to use NIV in these conditions, only do it where there is the option of intubating rapidly and safely — ideally ICU.

In a very small proportion of patients with these acute syndromes, respiratory function will dip just to a level where NIV is needed and then start to improve. For these patients NIV is clearly a much better option than intubation, tracheostomy and a protracted wean. The trouble is, how do you pick this sub-group out? You have a patient in front of you with deteriorating respiratory muscle weakness, but you have no idea how bad their worst point is going to be (Figure 39.1).

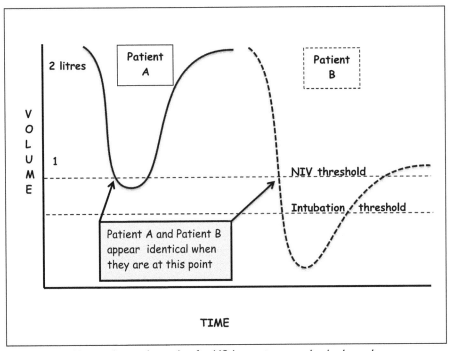

Figure 39.1 Alternative trajectories for VC in acute neurological syndromes.

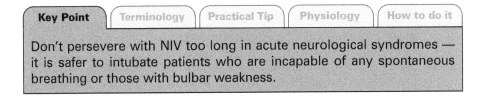

Key Point — Terminology — Practical Tip — Physiology — How to do it

Don't persevere with NIV too long in acute neurological syndromes — it is safer to intubate patients who are incapable of any spontaneous breathing or those with bulbar weakness.

Respiratory Monitoring

Looking at the patient is more important than the numbers generated by tests. You'll soon be able to spot those patients who are running into trouble, just by looking at how fast they breathe, which muscles they are using to breathe with and how much bigger (from the end of the bed) VC is than Vt. Watch tidal breathing, then ask the patient to take a really deep breath in. (Don't be fooled by spinal flexion and extension, without much expansion of the ribcage, during the VC manoeuvre.) You will learn not to be falsely reassured by reasonable test results in patients who are clearly running into trouble. Others may be poor at doing the tests, perhaps because they are very frightened, but your bedside assessment tells you (correctly) that they are fine for the moment.

The traditional way of monitoring respiratory function in acute neurological syndromes is to measure VC. If this falls below 1.5 litres, keep a closer eye on the patient and consider moving them to a critical care area. If it falls below 0.75 litres then you definitely need someone from ICU to take a look at them.

SNIP would be just as good as VC (see previous chapter) and easier for the patient. The meters for SNIP are smaller and cheaper than spirometers, but easier to lose at the back of store cupboards. Less than 20 cmH$_2$O is the SNIP threshold below which some form of ventilatory support is likely to be needed.

Peak flow meters are widely available. There is a good case for measuring cough peak flow rate in these patients along with VC. More than 300 l/min is fine, less than 150 l/min and it's time for an ICU opinion.

Measuring SpO$_2$ at the same time as these tests is easy. It starts to fall late on in the progression of muscle weakness.

Ventilator settings

Use pressure-control. You don't want the patient's failing respiratory muscles to have to do any work triggering the ventilator.

IPPV will give the best tidal volume, but use bi-level pressure- control (to help prevent basal atelectasis) if the SpO$_2$ remains low, or if you don't have the option of an exhalation valve.

Interfaces

An oro-nasal mask is the best option acutely. Once you have stabilised the situation, nasal pillows or a nasal mask are worth a try.

Cough-assist

Cough-assist devices (Chapter 43) may be really helpful for these patients. It can, however, be quite tiring for them and there is always the possibility that you will make the patient worse. Use cough-assist for short periods only, resting with NIV in-between.

Weaning

When you are weaning patients with obesity, scoliosis or COPD from ventilatory support, you can make a weaning plan and hopefully progress quite quickly. In neurological conditions the underlying disease may hold you back. If the diaphragm hasn't recovered, the patient will struggle with spontaneous breathing trials and you may have to put the weaning plan on hold.

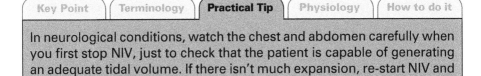

| Key Point | Terminology | **Practical Tip** | Physiology | How to do it |

In neurological conditions, watch the chest and abdomen carefully when you first stop NIV, just to check that the patient is capable of generating an adequate tidal volume. If there isn't much expansion, re-start NIV and try again at a later date.

Summary

- NIV helps some patients with acute neurological problems who develop type 2 respiratory failure, but most will need invasive ventilation
- Most of these patients will need NIV long term at home, often just at night
- Use pressure-control modes

40
Volume Modes

Learning points

By the end of this chapter you should be able to:

* **Define tidal volume**
* **Outline the difference between pressure- and volume-targeted NIV**
* **State the advantages of volume-targeted ventilation**
* **State the disadvantages of volume-targeted ventilation**

Up until now we have talked about target pressure: the same pressure is reached with each breath, but the amount of air entering the lungs with each breath (tidal volume) will vary — if the lungs are stiffer (less compliant), for the same pressure the tidal volume would become less (Figure 40.1):

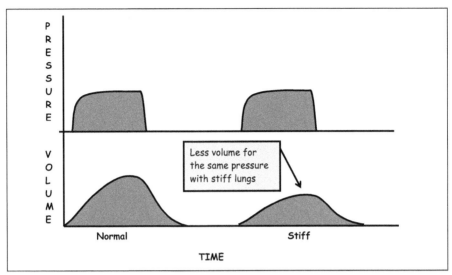

Figure 40.1 Effect of compliance on tidal volume. If the target pressure remains the same but the lungs become stiffer — the breath on the right — the tidal volume will be less.

In volume-targeted ventilation a target tidal volume is set, and the ventilator uses as much pressure as is necessary to get that amount of air into the lungs; if the lungs get stiffer, it uses a higher pressure (Figure 40.2):

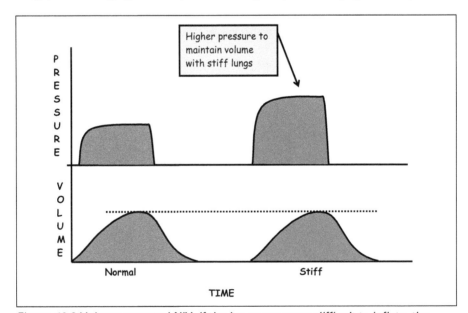

Figure 40.2 Volume-targeted NIV. If the lungs are more difficult to inflate, the ventilator uses more pressure to ensure that the target tidal volume is achieved.

Caution is needed in using volume-controlled ventilation in the presence of a pneumothorax or in patients with bullous lung disease, where high pressures could be a problem. However, the advantage of this arrangement is that you are more certain of getting enough air into the lungs. This is certainly the case in a "closed" system such as an ICU ventilator attached to an endotracheal tube; however, if there is a leak in the system, as there invariably is around the mask in NIV, the advantage of setting volume is less obvious, because some of the volume is lost through the leaks. The evidence in favour of either volume- or pressure-targeted ventilation is not convincing, but there may be an advantage in switching from one to the other if your patient is not improving. Volume-targeted ventilation has been used for many years to ventilate neuromuscular patients at home. It works very well. Although there is an overwhelming trend towards the use of pressure-targeted modes, we should not forget that there will still be some patients who would be better on volume-controlled ventilators. Longer-established NIV centres tend to have more patients with neuromuscular conditions and are more likely to use volume-targeted ventilators, for purely historical reasons.

"Smart" volume modes

Ventilator manufacturers have started to combine the advantages of pressure- and volume-targeted modes. One example is AVAPS (average volume-assured pressure-support). This is a servo mode of ventilation, whereby the ventilator alters what it does in response to changes in the patient's response. AVAPS tries to maintain tidal volume by increasing the inflation pressure. Another "smart" mode of ventilation is CS (for Cheyne-Stokes), which adapts to the cyclical changes in tidal volume and provides more pressure when the patient's effort reduces (Figure 40.3). The evidence so far is that these modes can provide more consistent ventilation. They seem to be well tolerated by patients. It remains to be seen whether in clinical practice there are substantial long-term benefits, or whether the greater sophistication compromises reliability.

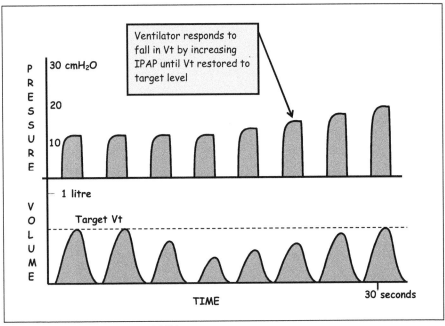

Figure 40.3 Volume-assured NIV.

Summary

- **Volume-controlled ventilation varies IPAP so that tidal volume is always the same**
- **Smart modes of pressure-controlled ventilation attempt the same thing**

41
Weaning to NIV from a Tracheostomy

Learning points

By the end of this chapter you should be able to:

• **Describe when and how to switch from tracheostomy ventilation to NIV**

Patients who have been intubated for any length of time often end up with a tracheostomy. How do we switch the ventilator support from invasive to non-invasive? First ask yourself if there is a reason why the tracheostomy should be left in place:

• **Are you sure there is no anatomical problem with the upper airway?**
• **Does the patient have a good cough?**
• **Is the sputum volume so high that it is going to be easier to suction through a tracheostomy?**
• **Are there bulbar problems which may make swallowing unsafe?**
• **Is the patient going to be ventilator-dependent 24 hours per day?**

Assess upper airway patency by letting the cuff of the tracheostomy tube down (with a fenestrated inner tube if this is an option), occluding the lumen and seeing if the patient can breathe. If they can't it may just be because there isn't much room around the tracheostomy tube. If in doubt, have a look with a fibre-optic scope.

You may need to change the tube to a more suitable one. Here are a few points about tracheostomy tubes:

- **A cuffed tube (Figure 41.1A) will protect against aspiration if bulbar function is impaired or if the patient has a poor cough reflex**
- **A cuffed tube provides a sealed system if the patient needs CPAP**
- **Even with the cuff deflated, it can be difficult for the patient to breathe around a tracheostomy tube through their own upper airway**
- **It is much easier to breathe around a smaller tracheostomy tube or an uncuffed tube**
- **Use an uncuffed tube (Figure 41.1B) if the tracheostomy is there only to allow suction of secretions from the bronchial tree**
- **A fenestration is a hole (or lots of small holes) half way up the tracheostomy tube, through which the patient can breathe**
- **Use a fenestrated tube (Figure 41.1C) when you want to block off the tracheostomy and get the patient to breathe through their upper airway**
- **With a fenestrated tube, you will need to use an inner tube without a fenestration when you put a suction catheter down to aspirate secretions**
- **Even with the cuff deflated and fenestration open, it can still be difficult to breathe through the upper airway**

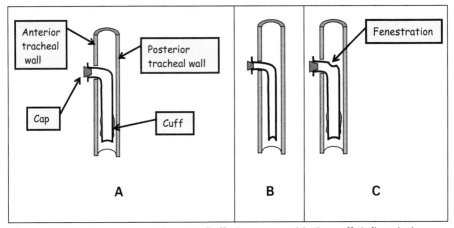

Figure 41.1 Tracheostomy tubes. A: Cuffed — even with the cuff deflated, there may be very little room for the patient to breathe around the tube. B: Uncuffed* — it is easier for the patient to breathe through their upper airway, particularly with a smaller diameter tube. C: Fenestrated — a hole allows communication with the upper airway; inner tubes come with and without fenestrations.

*fenestrated versions of uncuffed tubes are also available.

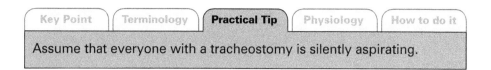

Key Point	Terminology	**Practical Tip**	Physiology	How to do it

Assume that everyone with a tracheostomy is silently aspirating.

Weaning failure

The psychology of weaning is very important. It is easy for a patient with a tracheostomy on ICU to get downhearted. A few things that can make a difference are as follows:

- Make them feel more human again by enabling them to speak
- See if it is possible for them to eat and drink
- Improve the night-time environment so they get some sleep
- Sit them out of bed
- Get them dressed in their own clothes
- Remove as many tubes and probes as you can
- A change of surroundings can work wonders; if you have the opportunity, move them from ICU to HDU or even a weaning centre

In the journey towards ventilatory independence, there will be ups and downs. So long as the general trend is in the right direction, you need to help the patients cope with the bad days. Every day you should have specific targets, agreed on by you and the patient. If the previous day was disappointing for them, don't be too ambitious the next day. If you and the patient both believe that you will get there in the end, then your chances of getting there are high. If "you" is a different person every day, it will not be so easy.

| Key Point | Terminology | Practical Tip | Physiology | **How to do it** |

Wean from a tracheostomy to NIV
- Select a nasal mask and check that it fits comfortably on the patient
- Connect the NIV ventilator that you are going to use to the tracheostomy and check that it is capable of ventilating the patient effectively
- Disconnect the ventilator from the tracheostomy and connect it to the mask
- Suction the trachea and pharynx
- Deflate the cuff
- Suction the trachea
- Occlude the tracheostomy and check that the patient can breathe around the tracheostomy tube. If not, change the tube for a smaller one. You could use a fenestrated tube, but this is not essential
- Attach the mask to the patient and commence NIV
- If the chest does not expand, increase the IPAP
- If the chest still does not expand, there is no connection between the upper airway and the lungs. Re-connect the ventilator to the tracheostomy. Think about examining the cords with a fibre-optic scope. Change the tracheostomy for a smaller one
- When the patient has been stable on NIV for 24 hours, remove the tracheostomy
- Occlude the hole by placing a dressing over it. Cover this with two long pieces of elastic adhesive bandage in an X, extending up over the clavicles. Don't use "sleek" — it will soon blow off
- If you are uneasy about removing the tracheostomy straight away, change it for a small cuffless tube

| Key Point | Terminology | **Practical Tip** | Physiology | How to do it |

Think about undiagnosed neuromuscular weakness in a patient who is struggling to wean.

Summary

- Make sure that the NIV ventilator is able to effectively ventilate the patient before you swap from a tracheostomy to NIV
- Use a small uncuffed tracheostomy tube during the transition

42
NIV as an Adjunct to Physiotherapy

Learning points

By the end of this chapter you should be able to:

- Describe when NIV can help with expectoration
- Select patients with bronchiectasis who are suitable for NIV at home
- Explain the difference between NIV and a cough-assist device

For many years, physiotherapists have used positive-pressure devices to help with chest physiotherapy. NIV is no different in principle. NIV ventilators can be used to inflate the lungs fully to prevent basal collapse (atelectasis), or to increase the volume of air inspired before a cough in order to aid expectoration. The main indications are post-operative use, bronchiectasis and neuromuscular problems.

Intermittent NIV post-operatively

Some patients may benefit from a short period of NIV every few hours or so in the immediate post-operative period. Expansion of the lung bases prevents atelectasis, with mobilisation and expectoration of secretions. This is not as an aid to weaning (Chapter 18), but the sorts of patients who may benefit will be similar:

- **COPD**
- **Obesity**
- **Scoliosis**
- **Neuromuscular disorders**

Patients with more severe disease who will be at increased risk of developing respiratory problems after surgery can be identified pre-operatively using spirometry and arterial blood gases.

Some operations are more likely to lead to respiratory complications:

- **Thoracic surgery**
- **Upper abdominal surgery**
- **Spinal surgery**

Prevention is better than cure, so planning to use NIV post-op in high risk patients who undergo high-risk procedures is more likely to succeed than waiting until the patient is in trouble.   An increasingly common indication for post-op NIV is after gastric surgery for obesity, where it has be shown to be safe and effective. As we've already noted, plan to use NIV post-operatively in an obese patient if they are likely to need opiates for analgesia.

Bronchiectasis

Evidence from studies in cystic fibrosis suggests that NIV is helpful in patients who desaturate during chest physiotherapy, in shortening the time it takes to recover from the physiotherapy session. It would seem reasonable to extrapolate this to bronchiectasis from other causes. It is unclear whether the volume of sputum expectorated is increased by the use of NIV.

NIV at night can help some patients with bronchiectasis. Their long-term survival is poor, but NIV can reduce hospitalisation and improve their quality of life. In younger patients, it may just get them through to a lung transplant. Consider nocturnal NIV in patients with bronchiectasis and the following:

- **Young age**
- **Severe disease**
- **Frequent hospitalisations**
- **Deteriorating blood gases despite optimal medical therapy**
- **Hypercapnia**
- **Symptoms of sleep disturbance**
- **Good tolerance of NIV**

The number of patients on long-term nocturnal NIV in your service is likely to remain pretty small.

Neuromuscular problems

NIV increases Vt. Inflation of the lower lobes of the lungs will be greater, which may prevent atelectasis. The prophylactic use of intermittent NIV in neuromuscular problems is debatable, but if the patient develops a chest infection then it can be very useful in conjunction with physiotherapy to aid expectoration of sputum.

NIV and rehabilitation

NIV can be used to help patients with COPD (and other respiratory diseases) to do some exercise and build up their peripheral muscle strength. The patient, or a helper, can carry a battery-powered portable ventilator. Alternatively, a mains-powered ventilator can be used with a treadmill or exercise bicycle.

Breath-stacking

If by NIV we mean anything other than the patient's own respiratory muscles producing ventilation, then we need to include breath-stacking, where the source of positive pressure is the physiotherapist or carer squeezing a self-inflating bag. We discussed this in Chapter 7. It is one of the easiest ways of getting some air behind a cough.

Glossopharyngeal breathing

Whilst we're on the subject of alternative ways of getting air into the lungs, there is the technique of glossopharyngeal or "frog" breathing, so called because you tend to look like a gulping frog whilst doing it. Basically the pharyngeal muscles force small gulps of air down into the lungs. Twenty or so small gulps make a decent sized breath. This can be used to supplement tidal breathing, or more commonly to help expectorate secretions.

Summary

- NIV can be used as an adjunct to chest physiotherapy, post-operatively or in bronchiectasis
- A small proportion of patients with bronchiectasis benefit from NIV at home

43
Cough-Assist Devices

Learning points

By the end of this chapter you should be able to:

* Describe the difference between a cough-assist device and a non-invasive ventilator
* Give an example of a patient who might need a cough-assist device

All the NIV we have discussed so far involves positive airway pressure. Cough-assist devices apply positive pressure during inspiration, but then switch to a negative airway pressure during expiration (Figure 43.1).

Key Point	Terminology	Practical Tip	Physiology	How to do it

Cough-assist devices use positive and negative pressure to help get secretions out of the lower respiratory tract.

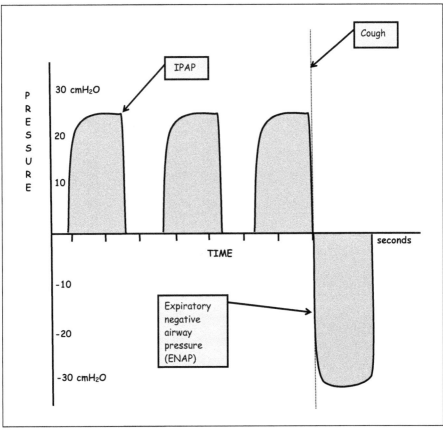

Figure 43.1 Cough-assist. After a few breaths with just IPAP, there is a rapid switch to expiration with a negative pressure applied to the airway.

The addition of expiratory negative airway pressure (ENAP) produces higher expiratory flow rates than with inspiratory positive pressure alone, which helps with expectoration of secretions. These devices work well in patients with severe respiratory muscle weakness, particularly if they develop a chest infection and are struggling to expectorate secretions. (Some patients who are already using nocturnal NIV find that stepping up their daytime use of NIV is all that is required during a chest infection, without the additional expense of a cough-assist machine.)

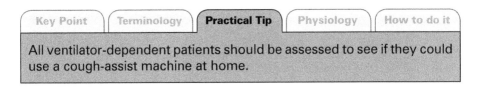

| Key Point | Terminology | **Practical Tip** | Physiology | How to do it |

All ventilator-dependent patients should be assessed to see if they could use a cough-assist machine at home.

Learning cough-assist is harder than NIV. It needs a real expert to teach the patient, and lots of practice. Using cough-assist every morning for a few minutes is the best way of maintaining proficiency in this technique, and clears any secretions that have accumulated overnight.

Key Point	Terminology	Practical Tip	Physiology	**How to do it**

Cough-assist
- Explain to the patient what a cough-assist machine is and why you want to try it with them
- Demonstrate the way it switches from positive to negative pressure
- Explain the point in the breathing cycle when you want them to cough
- Set the IPAP to the same as their current IPAP
- Set the ENAP to -30 cmH$_2$O
- Put the mask over their face
- Count five breaths in
- Then the patient coughs
- Take the mask off
- When the patient is ready, start another cycle
- Push up the IPAP and ENAP if the patient will tolerate it

Key Point	Terminology	Practical Tip	**Physiology**	How to do it

Cough
There are three phases of cough:

- Inspiration — the inspiratory muscles contract to get air into the lungs. This is important so that there is some air "behind" the cough
- Compression — the vocal cords close, then the expiratory muscles contract hard to generate a high positive intra-thoracic pressure
- Expulsion — after rapid vocal cord opening, the high intra-thoracic pressure results in really high expiratory flow rates, which then decay away

You will gather from this that an effective cough requires good function of the inspiratory, expiratory and vocal cord muscles (Figure 43.2).

cont ...

Key Point | Terminology | Practical Tip | **Physiology** | How to do it

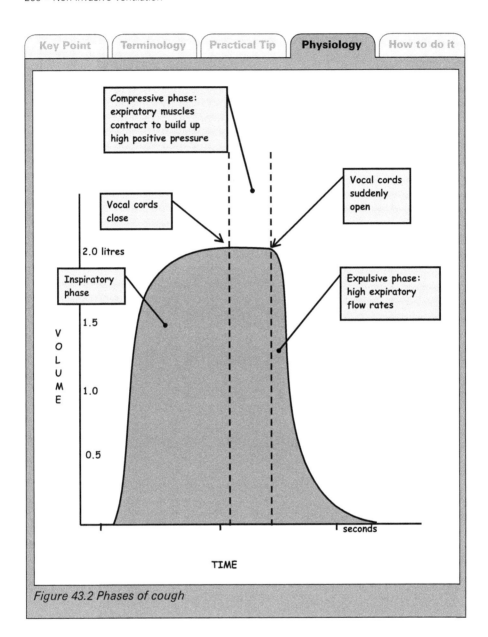

Figure 43.2 Phases of cough

Peak cough flow

A good way of assessing the effectiveness of a cough is to get the patient to cough into a peak flow meter. A peak cough flow of greater than 300 l/min implies that the cough is likely to be effective. Less than 150 l/min and the patient may not be able to clear secretions from their lower respiratory tract if they develop an infection. A simple peak flow meter connected to an oro-nasal mask will do the trick.

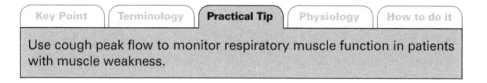

Key Point	Terminology	**Practical Tip**	Physiology	How to do it

Use cough peak flow to monitor respiratory muscle function in patients with muscle weakness.

Summary

- Cough-assist devices are good for helping patients expectorate
- They work best in neuromuscular conditions
- Patients who are 24-hour ventilator-dependent should have a cough-assist machine at home

44
Long-Term

Learning points

By the end of this chapter you should be able to:

- Give examples of the types of patient who use NIV at home
- Teach a patient the skills they need to set up their ventilator
- Discharge a patient home safely on NIV
- Plan their follow-up

Most of this book has been about acute NIV. We have strayed into some areas which are more relevant to the longer term. You may become interested in home NIV if you have a patient who presented in acute respiratory failure but is now better and needs to continue with NIV in the long term. You may have come across out-patients who are slipping into chronic respiratory failure and need to start NIV electively. Even if these patients go to a regional unit, you might like to know a little more, particularly if you are going to provide the local part of a "shared care" package.

Key Point	Terminology	Practical Tip	Physiology	How to do it

About half of the patients who use NIV long-term at home start this after an emergency admission to hospital with acute respiratory failure.

269

I am not going to cover all aspects of long-term NIV: there are several excellent books on the topic, details of which are in the bibliography. There is no one right way of setting up home NIV, and very little high quality evidence on which to base recommendations.

Patients

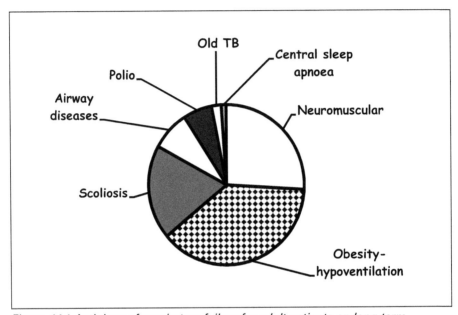

Figure 44.1 Aetiology of respiratory failure for adult patients on long-term ventilation in our unit.

Most home ventilation services have a large proportion of patients with either neuromuscular problems or obesity-hypoventilation syndrome (Figure 44.1). Smaller numbers of patients will have scoliosis. A few will have long-term sequelae of poliomyelitis or tuberculosis. There will be a handful of central sleep apnoea patients, and probably a cohort where the diagnosis is not entirely clear. The underlying diagnosis may not have been clear at the time your patient presented with acute respiratory failure, but over time, a clearer picture may emerge. There may be tests you can organise, or repeat, now that the patient is more stable. Over time you will accumulate a small group of patients who are undoubtedly helped by nocturnal NIV at home, but in whom it never really becomes clear what the underlying pathophysiology is. Keep an open mind.

The evidence base on which to make decisions about long term NIV in COPD is still evolving, which probably explains the wide variation in its use both within and between countries.

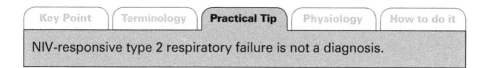

Key Point	Terminology	**Practical Tip**	Physiology	How to do it

NIV-responsive type 2 respiratory failure is not a diagnosis.

NIV competency

Get the patient to decide what they need to know about NIV. You can offer some choices and guidance, but it is much better if they make decisions about what they want to learn rather than you. Make a list and prioritise — start with the really important issues. You will be able to build on their knowledge and skills over time. The initial list for a patient with obesity-hypoventilation syndrome, for example, might be:

* What is wrong with my breathing?
* Why do I need a ventilator?
* How do I fit the mask?
* How do I turn the ventilator on?
* How do I keep the equipment clean?
* Who do I contact if I have a problem?

There are some key principles about any form of teaching:

* Active is better than passive learning — it is imperative that you get the person you are teaching to do things
* Assume nothing — it is easy to forget to explain something that is second nature to you, for example something simple like turning the ventilator on
* Less is more — don't teach too much in one session. Break things down into small manageable chunks
* Context/content/closure — explain why you need to teach the topic (for example, washing the mask), teach it, then summarise what has been learnt. Ideally the learner should do the summarising, which allows you to check that you have got the message across. This can be a bit depressing when they can't explain what you have so painstakingly taught them, but it is better to know that you have failed

Key Point | Terminology | Practical Tip | Physiology | **How to do it**

Teach a patient or carer a practical skill
- Explain what you are going to teach
- Explain why they need to know
- Demonstrate the skill, talking through each step along the way
- Demonstrate the skill again, but remain silent whilst you do so
- Perform the skill again, but this time in response to instructions from the patient/carer. If they give you the wrong instruction, don't carry it out; explain what the consequences would be if you did, then give the correct step. If you need to correct any instructions, you ought to repeat the whole skill again
- Get the patient/carer to demonstrate the skill to you. If they need prompts, repeat the whole skill one more time
- Document what you have taught

Key Point | Terminology | **Practical Tip** | Physiology | How to do it

Plan for everything that could possibly go wrong with NIV.

Equipment

Clearly the patient needs to know how to switch their ventilator on and off, and again be able to demonstrate this to you. It is unlikely that you will need the patient or their carers to adjust the ventilator settings at this stage, although some do when they are more conversant with NIV. Even if the ventilator allows you to lock the controls, it is good practice to write the settings down — keep one copy and put another in the folder the patient is going to take home with them.

Circuits have a habit of becoming disconnected from ventilators when they are moved around, so a diagram of what goes where is essential. In addition to being able to put on their mask properly, the patient needs to be able to take the mask apart for washing, and to re-assemble it. Cleanliness rather than sterility is the message for infection control at home. Equipment that looks clean is fine. Visibly dirty masks and circuits will be colonised by a variety of microorganisms, although surprisingly these seldom cause clinical infections. A daily wash in warm soapy water is best for masks, with a weekly wash in a dishwasher. Careful drying is important.

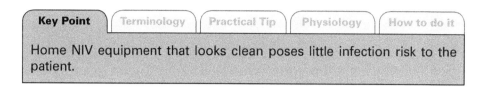

Key Point | Terminology | Practical Tip | Physiology | How to do it

Home NIV equipment that looks clean poses little infection risk to the patient.

Circuits should be cleaned about once every two weeks, ideally by putting them in an ordinary dishwasher. Alternatively, hot water and detergent can be used. The circuit should be disassembled into its component parts before washing, particularly the exhalation valve. It is important to hang the circuits up to dry thoroughly after washing. A weekly wipe down with a damp cloth or wipe will usually be sufficient to keep the ventilator clean.

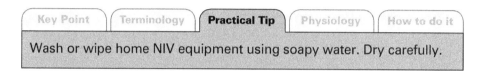

Key Point | Terminology | **Practical Tip** | Physiology | How to do it

Wash or wipe home NIV equipment using soapy water. Dry carefully.

You may also need to think about spare ventilators, back-up power supplies or a self-inflating resuscitation bag for emergencies in patients who are very dependent on NIV (see Chapter 45).

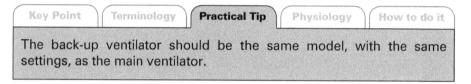

Key Point | Terminology | **Practical Tip** | Physiology | How to do it

The back-up ventilator should be the same model, with the same settings, as the main ventilator.

Written instructions

All the instructions need to be written down, for the patient or their carers to refer to when they are at home. You may choose to give them the instruction booklet for their ventilator, the leaflets that come with the masks and so on, but you need to summarise the important information. You could make up a folder for the patient with:

- A diagram of how to put the mask on
- Details of the type and size of mask, in case it needs replacing
- A diagram of how the circuit fits together
- Instructions for turning the ventilator on

cont ...

- A table of ventilator settings
- Action to take if the alarms go off
- An emergency contact number

Key Point	Terminology	**Practical Tip**	Physiology	How to do it

Have a dress-rehearsal in hospital. Get the patient into a side room and ask the carers who will be looking after them at home to deliver all the care in hospital for 24 hours. If there's a problem, hospital staff are on hand.

Follow-up

The longer the patient has been in hospital, the more stressful returning home is likely to be. In some cases it may be best to arrange a visit at home later that day. At the very minimum, a telephone call the next day will be needed, followed up by a home visit if necessary.

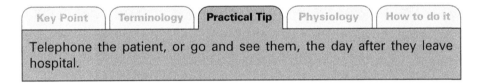

Key Point	Terminology	**Practical Tip**	Physiology	How to do it

Telephone the patient, or go and see them, the day after they leave hospital.

We usually see the patient at the hospital after one week, but a home visit would be better. They have another out-patient appointment in another month, and three-monthly thereafter. After a year, in very stable patients we sometimes push this interval up to 6 months. After another couple of years we may opt for annual appointments, provided the patient is happy with this and knows what to do if they have a problem.

The first follow-up visit

Ideally the first follow-up visit should be at home. If it is at the hospital, ask the patient to bring their ventilator with them. This may seem a bit over-the-top, but it is important that you check that they can assemble the circuit and attach their interface correctly.

It may seem obvious that the reason why the patient went into respiratory failure should be established, but it is easy to forget to do this if the patient came in with acute respiratory failure and was too unwell to have many tests done on admission.

Key Point	Terminology	**Practical Tip**	Physiology	How to do it

At the first follow-up visit, check that spirometry, mouth pressures etc. have all been documented, and that no other tests are needed to confirm what caused hypercapnic respiratory failure in the first place.

You will want to check their ventilator settings. If the arterial blood gases were abnormal at first presentation, check them again in the clinic. It is a good sign if daytime $PaCO_2$ is improving and the patient is sleeping well on NIV.

Key Point	Terminology	**Practical Tip**	Physiology	How to do it

If daytime $PaCO_2$ is improving, everything else is likely to be getting better as well.

Patients with neuromuscular weakness may feel better, look better and be sleeping better but still have a high daytime $PaCO_2$. This may just mean that they have such severe respiratory muscle weakness that they remain unable to maintain adequate alveolar ventilation, despite resting the respiratory muscles overnight. If the bicarbonate level is normal, it is highly likely that overnight, when the patient is on NIV, the $PaCO_2$ is much lower. You do, however, need to do a sleep study just to be sure.

Annual review

At the annual review, there are a few things to do:

- **Check for right-heart failure**
- **Check full blood count**
- **Service the ventilator**
- **Ask the patient to set up their NIV in front of you**

cont ...

- Check the emergency numbers
- Check arterial blood gases
- Arrange overnight monitoring, either routinely or only if there is a clinical concern, depending upon local practice
- Check any emergency procedures
- Has the patient become ventilator-dependent?

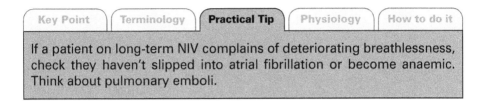

| Key Point | Terminology | **Practical Tip** | Physiology | How to do it |

If a patient on long-term NIV complains of deteriorating breathlessness, check they haven't slipped into atrial fibrillation or become anaemic. Think about pulmonary emboli.

Multi-disciplinary clinics

Depending upon the clinical condition and the stage at which the patient is, it may be desirable for your patient to see many different professionals. Clearly, making multiple trips to hospital is a bad way of doing this. Multi-disciplinary clinics are a good way of making this better, but they can be a bit intimidating. Having everyone else in separate rooms is good, if you have the space. In terms of efficiency, having motivated flexible colleagues in a clinic nearby is a good option.

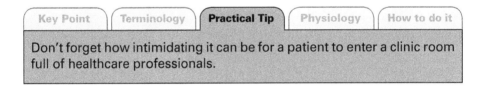

| Key Point | Terminology | **Practical Tip** | Physiology | How to do it |

Don't forget how intimidating it can be for a patient to enter a clinic room full of healthcare professionals.

Adolescent transition clinics

Transferring from paediatric to adult services can be a difficult time for the patient. If you are allowed to, use maturity rather than chronological age to decide when to swap over. If you can, set up a transitional clinic where they can see the paediatric and adult services together. When the patient has got to know the adult team (and understands the difference in how they will be able to access services), move them over to the adult clinic.

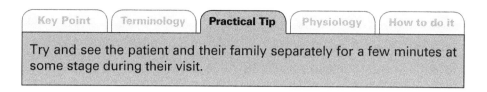

Try and see the patient and their family separately for a few minutes at some stage during their visit.

Adult emergency departments, acute medicine units and wards are pretty intimidating places for a youngster. It is much better to arrange direct access to a side ward on a ward where the staff know about NIV. You could show them round after one of their out-patient visits, so they know where they could be coming to if they were acutely unwell.

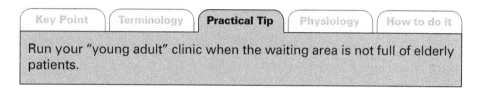

Run your "young adult" clinic when the waiting area is not full of elderly patients.

Summary

- Long-term NIV at home is an excellent treatment for patients with type 2 respiratory failure as a result of scoliosis, neuromuscular diseases or obesity
- Equipment used at home needs to be clean, rather than sterile
- Written instructions are good

45

The Ventilator-
Dependent Patient at
Home

Learning points

By the end of this chapter you should be able to:

*   **Give examples of different ways in which IPAP can be provided to a ventilator-dependent patient in an emergency**

There are a few extra safety arrangements you need to make if you are discharging a patient who is completely ventilator-dependent back into the community. If they can't manage more than a few minutes of spontaneous ventilation, your back-up systems need to be a bit tighter.

Key Point	Terminology	**Practical Tip**	Physiology	How to do it

In patients with progressive neurological diseases, check at each clinic visit that they can breathe spontaneously for at least 30 minutes. If they can't, you need to modify their NIV package.

Ventilators

The ventilator should have an internal battery, with an alarm that tells the carers that the mains power has failed. They should have a spare ventilator which is identical to the main ventilator, with the same settings. It is a good idea to rotate the two ventilators, perhaps daily, so that they know that both are in working order. It also means that their service history will be aligned.

Back-up power

Two ventilators with internal batteries will give quite a few hours of power, particularly if you heed the manufacturers' advice about running the batteries until they are flat before re-charging them. Nevertheless, it would be prudent to have an external battery to hand. A caravan or boat battery with a mains inverter is usually the cheapest option. In remote areas, some ventilator users choose to have a generator.

Self-inflating bag

A self-inflating resuscitation bag can be attached directly to the NIV mask for emergencies. It is a good option to have one in any case, to "bag" the patient if there is a medical crisis. If all else fails, "mouth-to-mask" ventilation would work.

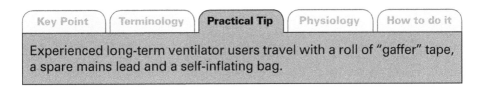

Key Point	Terminology	Practical Tip	Physiology	How to do it

Experienced long-term ventilator users travel with a roll of "gaffer" tape, a spare mains lead and a self-inflating bag.

Masks

One interface is seldom appropriate for 24-hour use. Rotating between oro-nasal masks, nasal pillows and mouthpieces will reduce the chances of pressure sores on the face. Eating, talking, reading, watching television, washing and sleeping may all need different interfaces.

Cough-assist

Any ventilator-dependent patient should be assessed to see if they would benefit from a cough-assist device at home. Some people struggle to use them, but long-term patients will often say that this is the thing that saved their life in a crisis. A daily cough-assist session, just to keep up-to-speed, is a good investment.

Safety

Long-term ventilator users experience equipment failure, on average, once every three years. This is sufficiently infrequent for you to be lulled into overlooking the risks. Rather like airline cabin crew going over and over safety briefings, even if you are a frequent flier, it is good practice to rehearse for emergencies on a regular basis. One of the team needs to go to the patient's home at least annually and be shown that the carers know what to do. This should be documented somewhere too.

Key Point	Terminology	Practical Tip	Physiology	**How to do it**

Check that home NIV is safe
- Explain to the patient and carers what you are going to do and why. Ask them to show you what they would do if:
- The ventilator starts to make strange noises and emit smoke
- The mains power of the whole house goes off, with no indication of how long it will take to fix
- Neither the main nor the spare ventilator are working
- The circuit splits
- The interface falls apart

Other things to check up on are the use of cough-assist, what the plan is if the patient develops a chest infection, who to call to arrange admission to hospital and who to contact for non-urgent advice or replacement equipment.

| Key Point | Terminology | Practical Tip | Physiology | How to do it |

Being at home is inherently risky if you are 24-hour ventilator- dependent, but spending the rest of your life in hospital isn't without its problems either.

It is much easier to get a ventilator-dependent patient home if there is one dedicated family member who is prepared to provide the majority of the care. Curiously, professional carers often need much more training than a family member before they are prepared to take on the same level of responsibility. The time it takes to train a team of carers rises exponentially with the number of people in the team.

Summary

- Being ventilator-dependent at home is inherently risky
- It requires careful planning
- It is better than being stuck in hospital
- A dedicated family member who can act as carer is crucial

Appendix 1

Bibliography

Disorders of Ventilation. John Shneerson. Blackwell Scientific Publications, Oxford 1988. ISBN 0-632-01668-X.

Noninvasive Mechanical Ventilation. John R. Bach. Hanley and Belfus, Philadelphia 2002. ISBN 1-56053-549-0.

Noninvasive Positive Pressure Ventilation: Principles and Applications. Nicholas S. Hill (ed.). Futura, New York 2001. ISBN 0-87993-459-X.

Non-Invasive Respiratory Support. A Practical Handbook. Anita K. Simmonds (ed.). Arnold, London 2001. ISBN 0-340-76259.

All You Really Need to Know to Interpret Arterial Blood Gases. Lawrence Martin. Lippincott, Williams and Wilkins, Philadelphia 1999. ISBN 0-683-30604-9.

Non-Invasive Ventilation and Weaning. Principles and Practice. Mark Elliott, Stefano Nava, Bernd Schonhofer (eds.). Hodder Arnold, London 2010. ISBN 9780340941522.

Appendix 2

List of key points

Key Point | Terminology | Practical Tip | Physiology | How to do it

CPAP applies positive pressure via a mask, but it does not provide ventilation.

NIV is all about getting the mask to fit well. (A mask that fits well today may not do so next week.)

More IPAP will usually mean more ventilation.

Kyphosis (antero-posterior curvature of the spine) is only rarely the explanation for why a patient has slipped into respiratory failure.

Patients with scoliosis who are hypercapnic need to be started on nocturnal NIV, irrespective of their pH.

When you start a patient with scoliosis or neuromuscular disease on NIV, set the ventilator rate to the patient's spontaneous breathing rate.

Pressure-control mode is the best mode of ventilation for most patients using NIV at home.

NIV masks are very different from oxygen masks — they fit much more tightly to the face in order to achieve a seal.

For long-term use at home, NIV masks and circuits that look clean are unlikely to be a source of infection.

Larger masks tend to increase dead-space.

In type 2 respiratory failure the $PaCO_2$ is elevated.

In respiratory acidosis, the $PaCO_2$ is greater than 6 kPa and the pH level is less than 7.35. If the bicarbonate is greater than 30 mmol/litre then the $PaCO_2$ has been high for some time — probably several days or more.

Type 2 respiratory failure is a failure of ventilation, hence non-invasive ventilation tends to work well. Type 1 respiratory failure is failure of oxygenation rather than ventilation, and NIV is less effective.

Hypoxia is much more dangerous than hypercapnia.

In MND, NIV works best for patients with symptomatic diaphragm weakness but well-preserved bulbar function.

In MND, accessory muscle recruitment at rest, or a respiratory rate >30 breaths per minute indicates that the patient is struggling to maintain adequate ventilation.

Hypercapnia is a late development in patients with respiratory muscle weakness. Start NIV straight away.

A pressure-targeted ventilator cannot deliver stacked breaths, unless you push up the IPAP.

In pressure-support NIV, the patient determines the respiratory rate and the duration of each breath.

Bi-level pressure-support is the most widely used mode for treating acute respiratory failure.

In a patient with a respiratory pump problem (skeletal deformity, reduced muscle power or reduced respiratory drive) an episode of hypercapnia, however transient, is likely to happen again, sooner rather than later.

In bi-level ventilation there is a small hole, or exhalation port, in the circuit near the mask to vent out exhaled air.

Patients using NIV at home tend not to get infections from dirty circuits. Their equipment needs to look clean, but it doesn't need to be sterile.

During NIV, bacteria do not spread into the circuit more than a few centimetres proximal to the expiratory port or valve.

If you want to get more air into the lungs, increase the IPAP.

IPAP should generally be between 10 and 30 cmH_2O.

In acute exacerbations of COPD, only use NIV in patients with a respiratory acidosis (pH <7.35)

The best results with NIV in COPD have used higher IPAP pressures. Aim for 30 cmH$_2$O if the patient will tolerate it.

Aim for an SpO$_2$ of 88-92% in COPD.

It will usually be apparent from checking arterial blood gases after about an hour of NIV whether or not it is going to work in acute respiratory failure.

Wean patients from NIV by lengthening their periods of spontaneous ventilation, not by reducing the NIV pressures.

Nocturnal NIV needs to be used for an average of more than four hours per night to do any good.

During pressure-support, the respiratory rate setting is the back-up rate, below which the ventilator will start to deliver breaths without being triggered.

Start nocturnal NIV in patients with a thoracoplasty if they are hypercapnic, irrespective of their pH.

In NIV the airway is not protected against aspiration.

Intubate the patient on the basis of their clinical condition, taking into account their arterial blood gas values — not on the blood gas values alone.

If you are going to use NIV post-operatively, start it as soon as possible after extubation — don't wait until the patient runs into trouble, as it is much less likely to be effective at that stage.

Patients with multiple fractured ribs do badly. Manage them on HDU and start NIV if they become hypercapnic.

Look at the patient first, then look at the ventilator: if the patient is not synchronising with the ventilator, then the numbers shown on the ventilator may be misleading.

If the patient is really sick, they need an arterial line.

If an alarm is not going to be acted upon, it should be disabled.

CPAP is as effective as NIV in acute LVF.

Nocturnal supplementary oxygen is better than NIV for most patients with chronic heart failure.

The diaphragm is the only respiratory muscle active during REM sleep. If it is weak or paralysed then it will be unable to maintain adequate ventilation during this phase of sleep.

The benefits of adjusting EPAP are much less than for IPAP.

If the vocal cords remain closed during a central apnoea, NIV will not be able to inflate the lungs.

Most modern ventilators use changes in the shape of the flow signal to decide when to trigger.

Adding supplementary oxygen into the NIV circuit can only increase FiO_2 to about 0.3 (or 30%).

Obese patients with chronic hypercapnic respiratory failure should be started on NIV, irrespective of the pH.

Obese patients with an elevated $PaCO_2$ are likely to need NIV at night in the long term.

Patients with OHS are at risk of underventilation if you put them on pressure-support, because of their poor respiratory drive.

If the difference between IPAP and EPAP is small, there will be little assistance to ventilation.

NIV is not mandatory for patients who develop respiratory failure at the end of their lives.

There is no legal duty to prolong life.

Withdrawing NIV does not mean giving up.

When you withdraw NIV at the end of life, it is the underlying disease that is the cause of death.

Respiratory depression from opiates and benzodiazepines at the end of life is minimal, and justified by their effectiveness in reducing breathlessness and distress.

Advance decisions to refuse treatment (ADRTs) are only of relevance when the patient no longer has the capacity to make decisions about their treatment.

When acting in the patient's best interests, rather than with their explicit consent, you must use whichever option is open to you that has the least restrictive effect on their liberty.

The first thing to do when looking at a patient on NIV is to watch carefully to check that the ventilator is synchronising with their own spontaneous respiratory efforts.

Most patient-ventilator asynchrony during sleep is caused by mask leakage.

With pressure-support, the I:E ratio setting only applies to back-up breaths.

If you are going to use NIV in type 1 respiratory failure, start it early.

In type 1 respiratory failure, use an NIV ventilator which has its own oxygen blender.

In type 1 respiratory failure, only use NIV in a critical care area.

There is always a danger of persevering with NIV too long. Don't delay intubation if it is apparent that NIV is not going to work.

Neck muscles are a last resort for breathing; we only use them at rest if the diaphragm and intercostals have failed.

Less than 10% of patients with myotonic dystrophy benefit from using NIV.

Don't persevere with NIV too long in acute neurological syndromes — it is safer to intubate patients who are incapable of any spontaneous breathing or those with bulbar weakness.

Cough-assist devices use positive and negative pressure to help get secretions out of the lower respiratory tract.

About half of the patients who use NIV long-term at home start this after an emergency admission to hospital with acute respiratory failure.

Home NIV equipment that looks clean poses little infection risk to the patient.

Being at home is inherently risky if you are 24-hour ventilator-dependent, but spending the rest of your life in hospital isn't without its problems either.

Appendix 3

List of practical tips

Key Point | Terminology | **Practical Tip** | Physiology | How to do it

Use a ventilator specifically designed for NIV.

Don't use lots of different types of ventilator. You'll struggle to keep everyone up to speed on how to use them. One for acute respiratory failure in hospital and a simpler one for long-term use at home are all you need.

Look at the patient to see if their chest is moving, before you look at the ventilator.

Always check on the ventilator display that the IPAP is reaching the pressure target you have set, particularly if there are lots of leaks.

Patients with scoliosis who have a VC under 50% predicted should have a clinical review and spirometry annually.

Many patients with severe scoliosis will underventilate for short periods during rapid eye movement (REM) sleep. You don't need to start NIV if the patient has no symptoms of sleep disturbance, but review the patient every 6 or 12 months and undertake a sleep study annually.

On many ventilators the respiratory rate is always referred to as the back-up rate. In pressure-control modes, this is the actual rate of ventilation, not just the back-up.

In acute respiratory failure in adults, start with a mask that covers the mouth and nose. In less acute situations, or in children, start with a nasal mask.

The lower straps on an NIV interface usually need to be much tighter than the upper straps.

Helmets work better for CPAP than NIV.

Watch out for lactic acidosis caused by too much nebulised salbutamol in a patient admitted with an acute exacerbation of COPD. Also, make sure that patients with diabetes mellitus stop their metformin when they are ill. Both these drugs are infrequent but important causes of metabolic acidosis.

Keep checking for fasciculation in the limb muscles of patients who present with isolated diaphragm paralysis, in case the underlying diagnosis is MND.

Respiratory failure is unlikely in MND if the VC is greater than 1.5 litres.

To assess the extent of respiratory muscle involvement in MND, just watch the patient breathing quietly. Then ask them to take a deep breath in. With experience, you will be able to spot those patients who are running into trouble, even if they can't do breathing tests.

In bulbar MND, if you try NIV it will become apparent fairly quickly if the patient is going to tolerate it.

MND is usually a rapidly progressive disease. Re-assess the goals of treatment regularly, and check that NIV is achieving them.

Every time a patient with MND attends clinic, check their VC, oxygen saturation and peak cough flow.

See patients with polio who are at risk of respiratory failure once a year in clinic. Ask about symptoms of nocturnal hypoventilation, frequency of chest infections etc. Look for right heart failure. Measure VC and check their arterial blood gases. Have a low threshold for doing overnight oximetry.

If you order oxygen for patients with chronic hypercapnic respiratory failure on NIV, tell the patient to use it only when they are on NIV at night and not during the day (when they are not on NIV). It is not like long-term oxygen therapy in COPD, which should be used for 12 or 15 hours per day. Supplementary oxygen without NIV can be dangerous in patients with chest wall problems, as in other causes of chronic type 2 respiratory failure, because it removes hypoxic drive.

If your patient's blood gases are not improving on bi-level NIV, always check that there is an expiratory port in the circuit and that it isn't blocked.

If the small bore pressure-monitoring and exhalation-valve tubes have been connected the wrong way round, you will hear lots of air whooshing out of the expiratory valve during inspiration.

If the exhalation port or valve is placed at the ventilator end of the circuit rather than the mask end, the patient will inevitably re-breathe only exhaled air. This is an easy mistake to make — always check the circuit.

Bi-level circuits sometimes have swivel connectors, safety valves (to allow the patient to breathe if the ventilator fails), pressure monitoring ports, oxygen connectors etc. It is easy to mistake these for an exhalation port.

When someone tells you that a patient is on "BIPAP 10 over 5", check whether they mean an inspiratory pressure of 10 or 15 cmH_2O. Sometimes the first number means the actual IPAP, or sometimes it means the amount over and above EPAP.

Very breathless patients may prefer a short rise time.

A high-dependency unit, with one nurse for two patients, is the best place to look after patients with an acute exacerbation of COPD requiring NIV.

Your NIV service needs to be able to cope with patients who need to start NIV in the Emergency Department and continue on it during transfer to another clinical area.

NIV ventilators designed for home use are OK for acute exacerbations of COPD, but a more sophisticated "HDU" ventilator with an integral oxygen blender will work much better.

The best place to add oxygen to an NIV circuit is just by the ventilator outlet. This is the simplest place to put it, and it allows the ventilator circuit to act as a reservoir for the oxygen during expiration.

Before you start to wean, establish effective ventilation (with a normal $PaCO_2$).

In patients with chronic lung disease, remember that their blood gases may be terrible even when they are stable and "well". If you aim for a normal PaO_2 it will take you ages to get them off ventilation.

Stopping nocturnal NIV is best done in one step, rather than cutting down the hours of use or reducing the ventilator settings.

After stopping nocturnal NIV, see the patient in clinic every week for three weeks and check their arterial blood gas.

Keep any patient with a thoracoplasty under annual review in your clinic.

In a patient who is not for intubation, beware of persevering with NIV for too long, past the point where there is any hope of the patient surviving.

Provided it is safe to do so, it is usually better to keep your NIV patients out of ICU. Staff in ICUs tend to feel more comfortable with invasive ventilation; the environment there can be pretty noisy; and day-night differentiation can be a problem for the patient's sleep clock.

Plan to use NIV immediately after extubation in an obese patient who is likely to need opiates for analgesia.

Extubate at a time of day when there is plenty of support at hand, when the patient can be rapidly intubated again if NIV fails.

Assume that everyone who has been ventilated for a few days or more is fluid overloaded. This will make it difficult to wean them, and they may develop pulmonary oedema (and therefore stiff lungs) when they are extubated.

Always consider the possibility of a pneumothorax if a patient with rib fractures deteriorates whilst on NIV.

If $PaCO_2$ is improving, everything else will probably get better in due course.

Wait at least 30 minutes after any change in ventilator settings before you check an arterial blood gas. If you have decreased IPAP or respiratory rate, it may take 60 minutes for the $PaCO_2$ to reach a stable state.

If you are using low pressure to detect ventilator disconnection, check that the alarm goes off when you remove the mask from the patient.

High flow is the most common reason for an NIV ventilator to alarm.

In acute LVF, start whichever you can get set up more quickly — either NIV or CPAP.

Transferring unstable patients on NIV is risky — are you sure it would not be better to intubate them?

If overnight oximetry shows an SpO_2 <90% for more than 30% of the night, it is quite likely that the patient will have daytime hypercapnia.

Keep patients with asymptomatic nocturnal hypoventilation under annual review if they have a disease which may deteriorate, for example progressive neuromuscular disease, polio or scoliosis.

If the bicarbonate level is elevated on a daytime arterial blood gas, but with a normal $PaCO_2$, do a sleep study to look for nocturnal hypoventilation.

In the absence of clinical pointers to a more generalised neurological disorder, neurological investigations have a pretty low yield in patients presenting with central sleep apnoea.

If you see a mixture of central and obstructive sleep apnoea on a sleep study, treat the obstructive part with CPAP and see what happens. Most of the time the central apnoeas cease to be much of a problem.

Use acetazolamide for a few days in patients with nocturnal hypoventilation and bicarbonate levels >35 mmol/l, whilst you get on top of their $PaCO_2$. This will reduce their bicarbonate pool and increase their responsiveness to CO_2.

Before you start adjusting trigger sensitivity, make sure that the mask fit is as good as you can get it.

Start NIV without supplemental oxygen and see what happens to the SpO_2. If it remains below 90%, try increasing the IPAP before you reach for the oxygen.

Choose between 88-92% and 94-98% as the target range for SpO_2, depending on the presence of underlying lung disease.

An obese patient with a normal daytime $PaCO_2$ but elevated bicarbonate is likely to have nocturnal hypoventilation.

If you're not sure if a patient has OSA or OHS, start them on NIV rather than CPAP. If it turns out to be mainly OSA, you can step them down to CPAP at a later stage.

Keep an eye out for overweight patients with COPD who are hypercapnic despite a reasonable FEV1 (> 50% predicted). They probably have OHS.

It is extremely rare for patients with OHS to lose enough weight to be able to stop using NIV.

In palliative care, always consider other options for helping breathlessness before resorting to NIV.

Agree a clear time frame with the patient when you plan to try NIV for relief of breathlessness or sleep disturbance, after which NIV will be stopped if the desired effect has not been achieved.

Withholding and withdrawing a treatment have the same legal status, but on the ground they feel very different.

Make sure that the HME is positioned in the circuit so that expired air passes through it.

If you use an HME filter in a ventilator-dependent patient, see what pressures and flows are reached when you take the mask off the patient. You may need to adjust your alarm settings to pick up disconnection.

When using a heated humidifier, there are no hard-and-fast rules about what temperature to set the heater at. To start with, set the thermostat in the middle of its range. The warmer it is, the more moisture the air will take up, but the patient may not like the heat on their face. (There is very little to be gained from an unheated water bath in the circuit.)

Adding a heated-wire humidifier may cause triggering problems during pressure-support.

Sort the mask out before you try anything else to improve synchronisation.

Switch to pressure-control if you can't easily correct triggering problems with pressure-support.

A low PF ratio is one of the things which predict failure of NIV in type 1 respiratory failure, particularly if it fails to improve quickly once you start NIV. The worse the problem with oxygenation, the less likely NIV is to work.

The commonest cause of patient-ventilator asynchrony is mask leak.

Many patients have incomplete lesions, involving mid-cervical segments in a patchy way. They will have some spontaneous ventilation, but it is easy to miss them slipping into ventilatory failure. Check their daytime bicarbonate level and do a sleep study.

Keep an eye on the VC of patients with incomplete or "medical" cervical cord lesions.

Think about undiagnosed neuromuscular weakness in patients who are struggling to wean from ventilation.

If the vital capacity (VC) of a patient with a neuromuscular problem is greater than 3.0 litres, the risk of them developing ventilatory failure is low.

Keep a close eye on patients with muscle diseases who have a VC <0.75 litres or an MIP <20 cmH$_2$O.

Daytime hypercapnia is a very late development in neuromuscular patients. Start NIV the same day (or make plans for palliative care).

Remember to do regular echocardiograms on patients with muscle conditions that may affect the heart: Duchenne, Becker, Emery-Dreifuss and limb-girdle (type 1b) muscular dystrophies.

Don't forget to arrange regular ECGs for patients with myotonic dystrophy, to check for conduction abnormalities.

Patients with neuromuscular problems have pretty compliant chests, so be careful not to overventilate them.

In neurological conditions, watch the chest and abdomen carefully when you first stop NIV, just to check that the patient is capable of generating an adequate tidal volume. If there isn't much expansion, re-start NIV and try again at a later date.

Assume that everyone with a tracheostomy is silently aspirating.

Think about undiagnosed neuromuscular weakness in a patient who is struggling to wean.

All ventilator-dependent patients should be assessed to see if they could use a cough-assist machine at home.

Use cough peak flow to monitor respiratory muscle function in patients with muscle weakness.

NIV-responsive type 2 respiratory failure is not a diagnosis.

Plan for everything that could possibly go wrong with NIV.

Wash or wipe home NIV equipment using soapy water. Dry carefully.

The back-up ventilator should be the same model, with the same settings, as the main ventilator.

Have a dress-rehearsal in hospital. Get the patient into a side room and ask the carers who will be looking after them at home to deliver all the care in hospital for 24 hours. If there's a problem, hospital staff are on hand.

Telephone the patient, or go and see them, the day after they leave hospital.

At the first follow-up visit, check that spirometry, mouth pressures etc. have all been documented, and that no other tests are needed to confirm what caused hypercapnic respiratory failure in the first place.

If daytime $PaCO_2$ is improving, everything else is likely to be getting better as well.

If a patient on long-term NIV complains of deteriorating breathlessness, check they haven't slipped into atrial fibrillation or become anaemic. Think about pulmonary emboli.

Don't forget how intimidating it can be for a patient to enter a clinic room full of healthcare professionals.

Try and see the patient and their family separately for a few minutes at some stage during their visit.

Run your "young adult" clinic when the waiting area is not full of elderly patients.

In patients with progressive neurological diseases, check at each clinic visit that they can breathe spontaneously for at least 30 minutes. If they can't, you need to modify their NIV package.

Experienced long-term ventilator users travel with a roll of "gaffer" tape, a spare mains lead and a self-inflating bag.

Appendix 4

Hydrogen ion concentration to pH conversion

H$^+$ (nmol/l)	pH
63	7.20
56	7.25
50	7.30
45	7.35
40	7.40
35	7.45
32	7.50

Appendix 5

kPa to mmHg conversion chart

kPa	mmHg
1	7.5
2	15
3	22.5
4	30
5	37.5
6	45
7	52.5
8	60
9	67.5
10	75
11	82.5
12	90
13	97.5
14	105
15	112.5
16	120
17	127.5
18	135
19	142.5
20	150

Index